Pit Boss Wood Pellet Grill & Smoker Cookbook for Athletes [4 Books in 1]

Plenty of Succulent High Protein Recipes to Godly Eat, Grow Muscle Mass and Feel More Energetic in a Meal

By

Chef Marcello Ruby

The trademarks used are without any consent, and the publication of the trademark is without permission or backing by the trademark owner. All trademarks and brands within this book are for clarifying purposes only and are owned by the owners themselves, not affiliated with this document.

Table of Contents

Pit Boss Wood Pellet Grill & Smoker Cookbook

INTRODUCTION 15

STRUCTURE 16

SMOKING.. 16

MONEY AND TIME SAVER.. 16

No need for firewood 17

Easy to clean 17

No stress on your back 17

COOK LIKE A CHEF AND IMPRESS THEM.. 18

HOW TO USE YOUR PIT BOSS WOOD PELLET GRILL?................. 20

VEGETABLE RECIPES 22

1. ROASTED FALL VEGETABLES 22
2. ROASTED PUMPKIN SEEDS... 23
3. WOOD PELLET COLD SMOKED CHEESE...................................... 25
4. WOOD PELLET SMOKED ASPARAGUS.. 26
5. WOOD PELLET GRILLED MEXICAN STREET CORN 28
6. CRISPY GARLIC POTATOES 30
7. GRILLED CORN WITH HONEY BUTTER.. 32
8. ROASTED PARMESAN CHEESE BROCCOLI................................. 33
9. SMOKED MUSHROOMS 34
10. CAJUN STYLE GRILLED CORN... 36
11. SMOKED BAKED BEANS 37
12. SPLIT PEA SOUP WITH MUSHROOMS 39
13. SMOKED BRUSSELS SPROUTS 41
14. ROASTED GREEN BEANS WITH BACON 42
15. STUFFED GRILLED ZUCCHINI 43
16. GRILLED ZUCCHINI 45

POULTRY RECIPES 47

17. WINGS.. 47
18. GRILLED CHICKEN... 48
19. SMOKED TURKEY BREAST 49
20. MINI TURDUCKEN ROULADE 50
21. HERB ROASTED TURKEY... 52

22. LEMON CHICKEN BREAST 54
23. APPLEWOOD-SMOKED WHOLE TURKEY 56
24. SPATCHCOCKED TURKEY 57
25. GARLIC PARMESAN CHICKEN WINGS 58
26. TRAGER SMOKED SPATCHCOCK TURKEY 60
27. GRILLED BUFFALO CHICKEN LEGS 61

BEEF, PORK & LAMB RECIPES 63

28. COUNTY RIBS 63
29. WOW-PORK TENDERLOIN 65
30. AWESOME PORK SHOULDER 67
31. PREMIUM SAUSAGE HASH 69
32. EXPLOSIVE SMOKY BACON 71
33. GRILLED LAMB BURGERS 74
34. LAMB CHOPS 76
35. LAMB RIBS RACK 78
36. LEG OF A LAMB 80
37. LAMB BREAST 82
38. NEW YORK STRIP 84
39. LAMB SHANK 85
40. SPICY PORK CHOPS 86
41. APPLE-SMOKED BACON 88
42. DELICIOUSLY SPICY RACK OF LAMB 89
43. GRILLED BUTTER BASTED RIB-EYE 90
44. PORK BELLY BURNT ENDS 92
45. SIMPLE GRILLED LAMB CHOPS 93
46. SMOKED SAUSAGES 95
47. WOOD PELLET SMOKED BEEF JERKY 96
48. BBQ BRISKET 98
49. BACON STUFFED SMOKED PORK LOIN 99
50. SMOKED BEEF RIBS 101
51. HERBED BEEF EYE FILLET 102
52. BEER HONEY STEAKS 104

FISH SEAFOOD RECIPES 106

53. SWEET HONEY SOY SMOKED SALMON 106
54. CRANBERRY LEMON SMOKED MACKEREL 108
55. CITRUSY SMOKED TUNA BELLY WITH SESAME ARO 111

56. SAVORY SMOKED TROUT WITH FENNEL AND BLACK PEPPER RUB 114
57. SWEET SMOKED SHRIMPS GARLIC BUTTER 116
58. SPICED SMOKED CRABS WITH LEMON GRASS 119
59. TEQUILA ORANGE MARINADE SMOKED LOBSTER 121
60. BEER BUTTER SMOKED CLAMS 124
61. BBQ OYSTERS 126
62. BLACKENED CATFISH 128
63. GRILLED SHRIMP 130
64. GRILLED LOBSTER TAIL 131
65. STUFFED SHRIMP TILAPIA 133
66. GRILLED SHRIMP KABOBS 135
67. WOOD PELLET GRILLED LOBSTER TAIL 136
68. BUTTERED CRAB LEGS 137
69. CITRUS SALMON 139
70. BARBECUED SCALLOPS 140

CONCLUSION 142

The Carnivore Meal Plan Cookbook for Athletes

INTRODUCTION **146**

CHAPTER 1: WHAT IS THE CARNIVORE DIET? **148**

1.1 HOW TO ORGANIZE YOUR MEAL PLAN FOR YOUR CARNIVORE DIET 149

1.2 15 DAYS MEAL PLAN FOR THE CARNIVORE DIET 152

1.3 WHAT FOOD IS INCLUDED IN THE CARNIVORE DIET? 157

1.4 WHAT FOOD ITEMS AVOIDED ON THE CARNIVORE DIET? 158

1.5 HOW CARNIVORE DIETS HAVE BENEFICIAL EFFECTS? 160

1.6 SIDE EFFECTS OF CARNIVORE DIET AND THEIR CURES? 166

CHAPTER 2: BREAKFAST RECIPES FOR THE CARNIVORE DIET **173**

1. Carnivore Breakfast Sandwich 173

2. Cheesy 3-Meat Breakfast Casserole Recipe 175

3. One-Pan Egg and Turkey Skillet Recipe 177

4. Keto and Carnivore Meatloaf Muffin 178

5. Carnivore Keto Burgers 180

6 Low-carb baked eggs 182

7. Spam and Eggs 184

CHAPTER 3: LUNCH RECIPES FOR CARNIVORE DIET 186

1. Carnivore Chicken Nuggets 186

2. Cheesy Air Fryer Meatballs 188

3. Scallops with Wrapped Bacon 190

4. Steak Tartare 191

5. Low-Carb Beef Bourguignon Stew 193

6. Lunch Meat Roll-Ups 198

7. Carnivore Braised Beef Shank 199

8. Herb Roasted Bone Marrow 202

CHAPTER 4: DESSERTS AND SNACK RECIPES FOR THE CARNIVORE

AIR FRYER COOKBOOK FOR TWO DIET 204

1. Bacony Carnivore Womelletes 204

2. Carnivore Cake 205

3. Egg Custard 207

4. Carnivore Chaffle Recipe 209

5. Meat Bagels 212

CHAPTER 5: DINNER RECIPES FOR THE CARNIVORE DIET 214

1. POT ROAST RECIPE WITH GRAVY 214

2. CARNIVORE SKILLET PEPPERONI PIZZA 217

3. CARNIVORE HAM AND CHEESE NOODLE SOUP 219

4. CARNIVORE MOUSSAKA 220

5. AIP CHICKEN BACON SAUTÉ 223

6. LOW CARB CARNITAS 225

7. CARNIVORE'S LASAGNA 227

CONCLUSION 231

Wood Pellet Smoker Grill Cookbook

INTRODUCTION   **236**

CHAPTER 1- WOOD PELLET SMOKER GRILLS   **238**

1.1   WHAT IS A PELLET SMOKER GRILL? 238
1.2   WORKING OF A PELLET SMOKER GRILL 239
1.3   BASIC COMPONENTS OF A WOOD PELLET SMOKER 240
1.4   USING YOUR WOOD PELLET SMOKER GRILL 244

CHAPTER 2-TRICKS AND TECHNIQUES   **250**

2.1   QUALITY MEAT AND SEASONINGS 250
2.2   USDA MINIMUM INTERNAL TEMPERATURES 251
2.3   GENERAL INFORMATION AND TIPS 254
2.4   SIMPLE TRICKS FOR BEGINNERS 258

CHAPTER 3-APPETIZERS RECIPES   **262**

3.1 ATOMIC BUFFALO TURDS 262
3.2 GARLIC PARMESAN WEDGES 263
3.3 BACON-WRAPPED ASPARAGUS 265
3.4 BOURBON BBQ SMOKED CHICKEN WINGS 265
3.5   BRISKET BAKED BEANS 268
3.6   CRABMEAT-STUFFED MUSHROOMS 269

3.7   HICKORY-SMOKED MOINK BALL SKEWERS 271
3.8   SMASHED POTATO CASSEROLE 272
3.9   ROASTED VEGETABLES 274
3.10   APPLEWOOD-SMOKED CHEESE 275
3.11   BACON CHEDDAR SLIDERS 276
3.12   TERIYAKI STEAK BITES 278

CHAPTER 4-LUNCH RECIPES   280

4.1   JAN'S GRILLED QUARTERS 280
4.2   CAJUN SPATCHCOCK CHICKEN 281
4.3   SMOKED PORK TENDERLOINS 282
4.4   PELLET GRILL SMOKEHOUSE BURGER 283
4.5   ROASTED LEG OF LAMB 285
4.6   TERIYAKI SMOKED DRUMSTICKS 286
4.7   APPLEWOOD WALNUT-CRUSTED RACK OF LAMB 287
4.8   HOT-SMOKED TERIYAKI TUNA 289
4.9   BAKED FRESH WILD SOCKEYE SALMON 289
4.10   BACON CORDON BLEU 290
4.11   PULLED HICKORY-SMOKED PORK BUTTS 292
4.12   PELLET GRILL PORK LOIN WITH SALSA VERDE 293

CHAPTER 5-DINNER RECIPES   296

5.1   ROASTED TUSCAN THIGHS 296
5.2   SMOKED BONE-IN TURKEY BREAST 297
5.3   CRAB-STUFFED LEMON CORNISH HENS 298
5.4   DOUBLE-SMOKED HAM 299
5.5   EASY NO-FAIL PELLET SMOKER RIBS 300
5.6   TEXAS-STYLE BRISKET FLAT 301
5.7   HICKORY-SMOKED PRIME RIB OF PORK 302
5.8   MEATY CHUCK SHORT RIBS 303
5.9   ROASTED DUCK À I' ORANGE 304
5.10   PETEIZZA MEATLOAF 306
5.11   SHRIMP-STUFFED TILAPIA 308
5.12   EASY SMOKED CHICKEN BREASTS 310

CONCLUSION   312

Air Fryer Cookbook for Two

INTRODUCTION: 316

CHAPTER 1: AIR FRYER BREAKFAST RECIPES 321

1. AIR FRYER BREAKFAST FRITTATA 321
2. AIR FRYER BANANA BREAD 322
3. EASY AIR FRYER OMELET 324
4. AIR-FRIED BREAKFAST BOMBS 325
5. AIR FRYER FRENCH TOAST 326
6. BREAKFAST POTATOES IN THE AIR FRYER 328
7. AIR FRYER BREAKFAST POCKETS 329
8. AIR FRYER SAUSAGE BREAKFAST CASSEROLE 331
9. BREAKFAST EGG ROLLS 333
10. AIR FRYER BREAKFAST CASSEROLE 336
11. AIR FRYER BREAKFAST SAUSAGE INGREDIENTS 338
12. WAKE UP AIR FRYER AVOCADO BOATS 338
12. AIR FRYER CINNAMON ROLLS 340
13. AIR-FRYER ALL-AMERICAN BREAKFAST DUMPLINGS 341

CHAPTER 2: AIR FRYER SEAFOOD RECIPE 343

1. AIR FRYER 'SHRIMP BOIL' 343
2. AIR FRYER FISH & CHIPS 344
3. AIR-FRYER SCALLOPS 345
4. AIR FRYER TILAPIA 346
5. AIR FRYER SALMON 348
6. BLACKENED FISH TACOS IN THE AIR FRYER 350
7. AIR FRYER COD 352
8. AIR FRYER MISO-GLAZED CHILEAN SEA BASS 354
9. AIR FRYER FISH TACOS 357
10. AIR FRYER SOUTHERN FRIED CATFISH 359
11. AIR FRYER LOBSTER TAILS WITH LEMON BUTTER 361
12. AIR FRYER CRAB CAKES WITH SPICY AIOLI + LEMON VINAIGRETTE 363

CHAPTER 3: AIR FRYER MEAT AND BEEF RECIPE 366

1. AIR FRYER STEAK 366
2. AIR-FRYER GROUND BEEF WELLINGTON 367
3. AIR-FRIED BURGERS 368

4. AIR FRYER MEATLOAF 370

5. AIR FRYER HAMBURGERS 372

6. AIR FRYER MEATLOAF 375

7. AIR FRYER BEEF KABOBS 376

8. AIR-FRIED BEEF AND VEGETABLE SKEWERS 377

9. AIR FRYER TACO CALZONES 379

10. AIR FRYER POT ROAST 380

CHAPTER 4: MIDNIGHT SNACKS 382

1. AIR FRYER ONION RINGS 382

2. AIR FRYER SWEET POTATO CHIPS 383

3. AIR FRYER TORTILLA CHIPS 384

4. AIR FRYER ZESTY CHICKEN WINGS 385

5. AIR FRYER SWEET POTATO FRIES 386

6. AIR FRYER CHURROS WITH CHOCOLATE SAUCE 386

7. WHOLE-WHEAT PIZZAS IN AN AIR FRYER 388

8. AIR-FRIED CORN DOG BITES 389

9. CRISPY VEGGIE QUESADILLAS IN AN AIR FRYER 390

10. AIR-FRIED CURRY CHICKPEAS 393

11. AIR FRY SHRIMP SPRING ROLLS WITH SWEET CHILI SAUCE 394

CHAPTER 5: DESSERT RECIPES 396

1. AIR FRYER MORES 396

2. EASY AIR FRYER BROWNIES 397

3. EASY AIR FRYER CHURROS 398

4. AIR FRYER SWEET APPLES 400

5. AIR FRYER PEAR CRISP FOR TWO 401

6. KETO CHOCOLATE CAKE – AIR FRYER RECIPE 402

CONCLUSION: 404

Pit Boss Wood Pellet Grill & Smoker Cookbook

70+ Succulent Summer Recipes to Eat Well, Feel more Energetic, and Amaze Them

By

Chef Marcello Ruby

Table of Contents

INTRODUCTION 15

STRUCTURE 16
SMOKING 16
MONEY AND TIME SAVER 16
No need for firewood 17
Easy to clean 17
No stress on your back 17
COOK LIKE A CHEF AND IMPRESS THEM 18
HOW TO USE YOUR PIT BOSS WOOD PELLET GRILL? 20

VEGETABLE RECIPES 22

1.   ROASTED FALL VEGETABLES 22
2.   ROASTED PUMPKIN SEEDS 23
3.   WOOD PELLET COLD SMOKED CHEESE 25
4.   WOOD PELLET SMOKED ASPARAGUS 26
5.   WOOD PELLET GRILLED MEXICAN STREET CORN 28
6.   CRISPY GARLIC POTATOES 30
7.   GRILLED CORN WITH HONEY BUTTER 32
8.   ROASTED PARMESAN CHEESE BROCCOLI 33
9.   SMOKED MUSHROOMS 34
10. CAJUN STYLE GRILLED CORN 36
11. SMOKED BAKED BEANS 37
12. SPLIT PEA SOUP WITH MUSHROOMS 39
13. SMOKED BRUSSELS SPROUTS 41
14. ROASTED GREEN BEANS WITH BACON 42
15. STUFFED GRILLED ZUCCHINI 43
16. GRILLED ZUCCHINI 45

POULTRY RECIPES 47

17. WINGS 47
18. GRILLED CHICKEN 48
19. SMOKED TURKEY BREAST 49
20. MINI TURDUCKEN ROULADE 50
21. HERB ROASTED TURKEY 52
22. LEMON CHICKEN BREAST 54
23. APPLEWOOD-SMOKED WHOLE TURKEY 56
24. SPATCHCOCKED TURKEY 57
25. GARLIC PARMESAN CHICKEN WINGS 58
26. TRAGER SMOKED SPATCHCOCK TURKEY 60
27. GRILLED BUFFALO CHICKEN LEGS 61

BEEF, PORK & LAMB RECIPES 63

28. COUNTY RIBS 63
29. WOW-PORK TENDERLOIN 65
30. AWESOME PORK SHOULDER 67
31. PREMIUM SAUSAGE HASH 69

32. EXPLOSIVE SMOKY BACON...71
33. GRILLED LAMB BURGERS..74
34. LAMB CHOPS..76
35. LAMB RIBS RACK...78
36. LEG OF A LAMB..80
37. LAMB BREAST..82
38. NEW YORK STRIP...84
39. LAMB SHANK...85
40. SPICY PORK CHOPS...86
41. APPLE-SMOKED BACON...88
42. DELICIOUSLY SPICY RACK OF LAMB...89
43. GRILLED BUTTER BASTED RIB-EYE..90
44. PORK BELLY BURNT ENDS..92
45. SIMPLE GRILLED LAMB CHOPS..93
46. SMOKED SAUSAGES..95
47. WOOD PELLET SMOKED BEEF JERKY..96
48. BBQ BRISKET..98
49. BACON STUFFED SMOKED PORK LOIN...99
50. SMOKED BEEF RIBS..101
51. HERBED BEEF EYE FILLET..102
52. BEER HONEY STEAKS...104

FISH SEAFOOD RECIPES..106

53. SWEET HONEY SOY SMOKED SALMON...106
54. CRANBERRY LEMON SMOKED MACKEREL...108
55. CITRUSY SMOKED TUNA BELLY WITH SESAME ARO...111
56. SAVORY SMOKED TROUT WITH FENNEL AND BLACK PEPPER RUB..............................114
57. SWEET SMOKED SHRIMPS GARLIC BUTTER..116
58. SPICED SMOKED CRABS WITH LEMON GRASS..119
59. TEQUILA ORANGE MARINADE SMOKED LOBSTER..121
60. BEER BUTTER SMOKED CLAMS..124
61. BBQ OYSTERS...126
62. BLACKENED CATFISH...128
63. GRILLED SHRIMP..130
64. GRILLED LOBSTER TAIL..131
65. STUFFED SHRIMP TILAPIA..133
66. GRILLED SHRIMP KABOBS...135
67. WOOD PELLET GRILLED LOBSTER TAIL..136
68. BUTTERED CRAB LEGS..137
69. CITRUS SALMON...139
70. BARBECUED SCALLOPS..140

CONCLUSION..142

Introduction

Pit Boss Wood Pellet Smoker Grill is one of our newest outdoor grills and smoker combos. It has it all: the ultimate cooking environment, a compact footprint, and an unbeatable price. Its ability to smoke and grill is unmatched, with the capacity to grill for up to 700 guests. So if you've been looking for the perfect smoker/grill combo but could not find one that had all the features you wanted, search no more.

Pit Boss Wood Pellet Smoker Grill has many features that make it stand out from other models on our site.

This grill is the best value you can find on the market for a smoking and grilling combo. It's perfect for those who need space or budget constraints. Pit Boss has two side shelves that fold up when not in use, leaving more space to cook when needed. It also has a fold-down warming rack, so you can cook more without having to open up your pit early. You can put it on the side of your house or in your garage and still have plenty of room to store other things.

Pit Boss is also a multi-fuel grill, meaning you can switch from wood to charcoal in under 10 minutes. It comes with everything you need to start smoking right out of the box. You don't have to worry about temperatures or knowing which wood pellets work best for certain kinds of meat, like other wood pellet smokers. That's because Pit Boss comes with their patented cook control system that lets you set precise temperature thresholds and wood pellet ratios for your grilling needs.

Pit Boss has a large 640 sq. in. total cooking area and an additional 640 sq. in. warming rack, in addition to thick, double-walled legs that are specifically designed for outdoor cooking. The thick stainless steel walls are durable and strong enough to withstand the harshest conditions and use while still looking great at your home or cabin! The legs have a channeled bottom for safe smoking under any weather conditions, including rain or snow.

The front and top racks of this grill provide you with a total of 680 sq. in. of cooking space! That is very close to the 700 sq. in.

Structure

Pit Boss Wood Pellet Smoker Grill looks great in any outdoor setting. The stainless steel legs and double-walled body also have an attractive black powder-coated steel hood with a grease cup. Because this is a wood pellet smoker, it can smoke well over 10 hours at a time without adding more fuel. It also has one of the most durable, high-quality knobs on the market.

Smoking

When you're ready to start smoking, Pit Boss will provide you with more than enough power for your grilling needs. It boasts an impressive 2,500 sq. in. cooking space, including two 675 sq. in. cooking grates and two upper and lower vents, letting you smoke for up to 4 hours at a time!

It also gives you a total of 13 pre-set temperature settings that you can easily adjust to your needs. This grill has an automatic self-cleaning feature, so your cooking space will always be ready for another cookout! You'll also be able to monitor the internal temperature of your food with the thermometer on the door.

There are many grilling accessories available that can make your Pit Boss Wood Pellet Smoker Grill even more versatile and useful, without all the extra expense of buying separate tools or accessories.

Money and Time Saver

The tool you need to save money and time is right here!

No need to spend money on expensive wood pellets when these will last longer than you can imagine. No need to spend time chopping wood or looking for the right kind of wood. These are easy to use, durable, and affordable in comparison to other types of pellets. You won't be going back to charcoal anytime soon after using these! :)

From start to finish, your grill is ready for cooking! The filter cup makes filling and cleaning the hopper a breeze, and since it holds up to a full 60 lbs. of pellets at once, you won't have to worry about running out in the middle of grilling season.

Pit Boss offers a frying pan accessory for this grill, which you can add to your package for an amazing price of $19.99 - that means you already have a grill and a smoker! This frying pan is made from cast iron to make sure that whatever you fry stays crisp and delicious. It also comes with a convenient drain hole at the bottom of the pan to help collect unwanted grease for easy disposal.

No need for firewood

You can use this independently, without firewood. All the fuel you need is contained within the grill.

This grill saves energy costs because there is no need for added gas or charcoal. The only thing you have to do is to plug it in

When you are hosting a party, this is a good alternative to the traditional grills. It can cook a larger quantity of food, save time and money by not having a long cooking session.

Easy to clean

Just wipe the grease and use soap for a quick clean. You can have it as clean as new in minutes.

This is the best feature of this grill. It has heavy-duty mesh, which allows for an easier cleaning process.

It does not rust either. Stainless steel grill is a good alternative to stainless steel appliances, and it will last longer because of the heavy-duty mesh.

No stress on your back

Since you need to do nothing but walk away while the greasewood pellet cooker cooks your food, you can spend more time socializing or doing other things without worrying about firewood or gas grill running out of fuel or charcoal as these tend to happen quite frequently, especially if you are hosting a barbecue party with a traditional charcoal or gas grill at your home. This high-efficiency pellet wood smoke cooker takes care of all these problems.

You don't have to buy firewood which saves you money over time. They can last for years, and you can be assured of consistent heat. It is easy to maintain, and on top of all that, it doesn't require much skill to use. This grill will save you a lot of trouble during those busy summer nights when your friends are over, allowing you more time with them

If anything is holding back this grill from being perfect, It's the size.

Cook like a chef and impress them

The Pit Boss Wood Pellet Smoker Grill will allow you to smoke, grill, and bake with the best cooking tools available. You will be able to easily make the perfect barbecue meats, deliciously done fish and seafood, and so much more!

Get everything you need in one unit. The Pit Boss Wood Pellet Smoker Grill has all of your smoking needs covered with plenty of room for grilling when not in use.

Have friends over or corporate events at your place? The large cooking area on this smoker grill makes it easy to cook a larger quantity of food at one time. No more "scrounging around," looking for a place on your outdoor grill to make extra food. You can cook your main dish and sides simultaneously, with no extra effort on your part. This saves you time and money!

No need to worry about the weather conditions while you're cooking. The Pit Boss Wood Pellet Smoker Grill is built from durable materials that will withstand all types of weather conditions so that you can enjoy grilling and smoking no matter what Mother Nature throws your way.

Everything needed in one unit Extra large cooking area for main dishes, sides, extras Large capacity holds up to 60 lbs.

Get the same results using less wood. The Pit Boss Wood Pellet Smoker Grill has an adjustable air control system that allows you to control the air intake and help regulate how much wood is going through the unit at one time. This controls how much heat you put out, as well as how many pellets are going through the unit at any given time, saving you money and helping you get a great smoke flavor!

Besides, the bottom warming rack holds up to 20 lbs of food, great for entertaining. The fold-down warming rack is great when cooking large items like whole chickens or fish.

Impress them with the perfect BBQ grilling recipe for your family, friends, or co-workers. Our Pit Boss Wood Pellet Grill is the ultimate easy-to-use outdoor cooking grill that will deliver your food with unparalleled convenience and flavour.

Our smart grill is loaded with high-tech features that help you get the precise results you want. The built-in meat probe and side shelf allow all of your food to be cooked evenly without babysitting the grill; the food sensor display lets you know when your meat has reached its internal temperature. These great features combine to make grilling even easier.

The single most important aspect of a BBQ grill when cooking outdoors is efficiency — your fuel should last as long as possible to reduce time spent refuelling and clean-up between cooks. That's why Pit Boss designed our pit grill to burn wood pellets as fuel, eliminating the need for messy propane canisters.

You'll also love the starter set, designed to provide you with everything you need to start grilling immediately. The 36" x 18" cast iron cooking grates are heavy and made of premium materials, while the side shelves are a convenient spot for your hot coals and grill tools. The cast iron drip pan is perfect for collecting drippings and leftovers.

Unlike most pellet grills on the market, our Pit Boss wood pellet grill uses one of the finest available wood-burning grills. We use only premium quality hardwood to create a combustion chamber where high-quality pellets burn cleanly and efficiently. Besides, we use specialized venturi-assisted opening valves that supplement airflow, making your food taste even better when cooked on our pit grill.

How to Use Your Pit Boss Wood Pellet Grill?

Pellet grills are high-tech machines that are powered by a motor connected to an auger system, where wood pellets are dropped into an enclosed area and then distributed evenly over hot coals. A digital controller regulates temperature by turning the drill on or off as necessary to maintain steady temperatures throughout the cooking process. A thermostat attached to the drill regulates the final temperature. Propane and charcoal are also delivered through a tube into a chamber to supply additional heat. A hopper on top of the drill delivers pellets when needed. The standard drill operates at a maximum speed of about 200 to 210 pounds per hour at temps between 180 and 200 degrees, depending on the type of pellets used.

This grill is easy to use, easy to clean up, and looks great. It comes with a large cooking area and a hopper that feeds the pellets into the grill continuously. The best part about using this grill is that you do not need to mess with any gas or charcoal because there is no open flame. You just plug it in, turn it on, and let it cook.

The Pit Boss 700 also comes with a meat probe that measures its temperature while it cooks. This feature allows you to leave once you are done cooking, so you don't have to sacrifice time to sit there and watch your food cook.

The benefit of using wood pellets is that they do not have smoke points, or what is commonly referred to as juiciness, leading to more even cooking temperatures and fewer flare-ups at all times during the smoking process. The low smoke point also makes them ideal for cooking with smaller amounts of meat because it will take longer for your meat to be fully cooked before it burns and tastes burnt.

The top of the grill has a pan for grilling and an assortment of cooking racks. It comes with one oil drip pan, and a grease drip pan placed just below the cooking grates. There is also a drip tray above the grease drip pan. That brings me to the next benefit of this grill, the grease container located on top of your food inside the grill. This eliminates all that excess grease that normally builds up around the edges because now your food will not sit in it. The flavor from all those juices will also be retained due to this grill's large cooking area, which keeps your meat tasting fresh and well-seasoned rather than dry and crunchy (which is what happens when cooking over direct heat).

Vegetable Recipes

1. Roasted Fall Vegetables

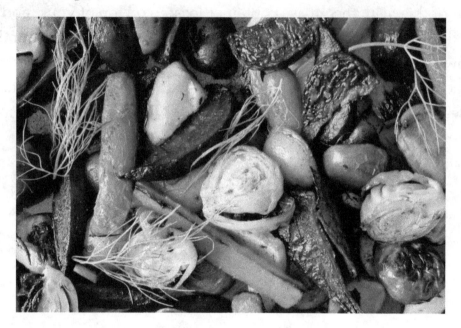

Preparation Time: 10 minutes

Cooking Time: 35 minutes

Servings: 8

Ingredients:

- Potatoes – ½ pound

- Brussels sprouts, halved – ½ pound

- Butternut squash, dice – ½ pound

- Cremini mushrooms, halved – 1 pint

- Salt – 1 tablespoon

- Ground black pepper – ¾ tablespoon

- Olive oil – 2 tablespoons

Directions:

1. In the meantime, take a large bowl, place potatoes in it, add salt and black pepper, drizzle with oil and then toss until coated.

2. Take a sheet tray and then spread seasoned potatoes on it.

3. When the grill has preheated, place a sheet pan containing potatoes on the grilling rack and then grill for 15 minutes.

4. Then add mushrooms, sprouts into the pan, toss to coat, and then continue grilling for 20 minutes until all the vegetables have turned nicely browned and thoroughly cooked.

5. Serve immediately.

Nutrition:

- Calories: 80 Carbs: 7g
- Fat: 6g Protein: 1g

2. **Roasted Pumpkin Seeds**

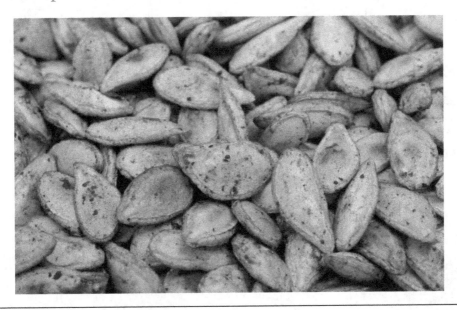

Preparation Time: 10 minutes

Cooking Time: 40 minutes

Servings: 8

Ingredients:

Pumpkin seeds – 1 pound

Salt – 1 tablespoon

Olive oil – 1 tablespoon

Directions:

1. In the meantime, take a baking sheet, grease it with oil, spread pumpkin seeds on it and then stir until coated.

2. When the grill has preheated, place a baking sheet containing pumpkin on the grilling rack and let grill for 20 minutes.

3. Season pumpkin seeds with salt, switch the grill temperature to 325 degrees F and continue grilling for 20 minutes until roasted.

4. When done, let pumpkin seeds cool slightly and then serve.

Nutrition:

- Calories: 130
- Carbs: 13g
- Fat: 5g
- Protein 8g

3. Wood Pellet Cold Smoked Cheese

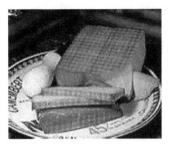

Preparation Time: 5 minutes

Cooking Time: 2 minutes

Servings: 10

Ingredients:

- Ice

- One aluminum pan, full-size and disposable

- One aluminum pan, half-size, and disposable

- Toothpicks

- A block of cheese

Directions:

1. Preheat the wood pellet to 165°F with the lid closed for 15 minutes.

2. Place the small pan in the large pan. Fill the surrounding of the small pan with ice.

3. Place the cheese in the small pan on top of toothpicks, then place the pan on the grill and close the lid.

4. Smoke cheese for 1 hour, flip the cheese, and smoke for one more hour with the lid closed.

5. Remove the cheese from the grill and wrap it in parchment paper. Store in the fridge for 2 3 days for the smoke flavor to mellow.

6. Remove from the fridge and serve. Enjoy.

Nutrition:

Calories: 1910

Total Fat: 7g

Saturated Fat: 6g

Total Carbs: 2g

Net Carbs: 2g

Protein: 6g

Sugar: 1g

Fiber: 0g

Sodium: 340mg

Potassium: 0mg

4. Wood Pellet Smoked Asparagus

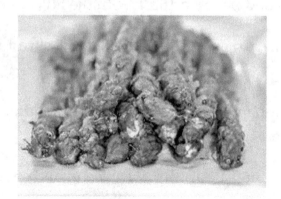

Preparation Time: 5 minutes

Cooking Time: 1 hour

Servings: 4

Ingredients:

- One bunch of fresh asparagus ends cut

- 2 tbsp. olive oil

- Salt and pepper to taste

Directions:

1. Fire up your wood pellet smoker to 230°F

2. Place the asparagus in a mixing bowl and drizzle with olive oil. Season with salt and pepper.

3. Place the asparagus in a tinfoil sheet and fold the sides such that you create a basket.

4. Smoke the asparagus for 1 hour or until soft, turning after half an hour.

5. Remove from the grill and serve. Enjoy.

Nutrition:

Calories: 43

Total Fat: 2g

Total Carbs: 4g

Net Carbs: 2g

Protein: 3g

Sugar: 2g

Fiber: 2g

Sodium: 148mg

5. Wood Pellet Grilled Mexican Street Corn

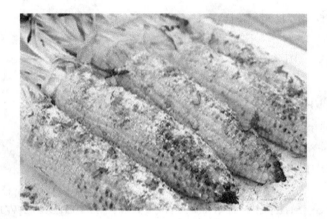

Preparation Time: 5 minutes

Cooking Time: 25 minutes

Servings: 6

Ingredients:

- Six ears of corn on the cob

- 1 tbsp. olive oil

- Kosher salt and pepper to taste

- 1/4 cup mayo

- 1/4 cup sour cream

- 1 tbsp. garlic paste

- 1/2 tbsp. chili powder

- Pinch of ground red pepper

- 1/2 cup coria cheese, crumbled

- 1/4 cup cilantro, chopped

- Six lime wedges

Directions:

1. Brush the corn with oil.

2. Sprinkle with salt.

3. Place the corn on a wood pellet grill set at 350°F. Cook for 25 minutes as you turn it occasionally.

4. Meanwhile, mix mayo, cream, garlic, chili, and red pepper until well combined.

5. Let it rest for some minutes, then brush with the mayo mixture.

6. Sprinkle cottage cheese, more chili powder, and cilantro. Serve with lime wedges. Enjoy.

Nutrition:

Calories: 144

Total Fat: 5g

Saturated Fat: 2g

Total Carbs: 10g

Net Carbs: 10g

Protein: 0g

Sugar: 0g

Fiber: 0g

Sodium: 136mg

Potassium: 173mg

6. Crispy Garlic Potatoes

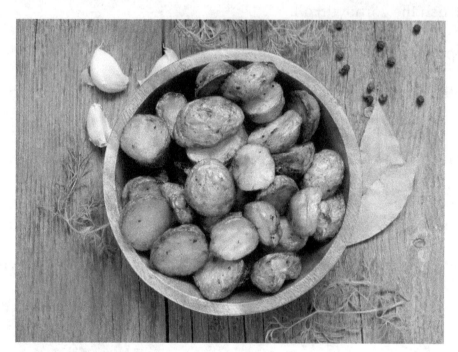

Preparation Time: 15 minutes

Cooking Time: 40 minutes

Servings: 4

Ingredients:

- Baby potatoes, scrubbed – 1 pound

- Large white onion, peeled, sliced – 1

- Garlic, peeled, sliced – 3

- Chopped parsley – 1 teaspoon

- Butter, unsalted, sliced – 3 tablespoons

Directions:

1. In the meantime, cut potatoes in slices and then arrange them on a large piece of foil or baking sheet, separating potatoes by onion slices and butter.

2. Sprinkle garlic slices over vegetables, and then season with salt, black pepper, and parsley.

3. When the grill has preheated, place a baking sheet containing potato mixture on the grilling rack and grill for 40 minutes until potato slices have turned tender.

4. Serve immediately.

Nutrition:

- Calories: 150
- Carbs: 15g
- Fat: 10g
- Protein: 1g

7. Grilled Corn With Honey Butter

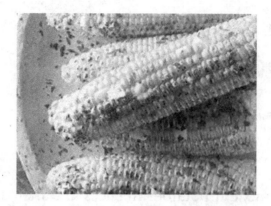

Servings: 6

Cooking Time: 10 Minutes

Ingredients:

- 6 pieces corn, husked

- 2 tablespoons olive oil

- Salt and pepper to taste

- ½ cup butter, room temperature

- ½ cup honey

Directions:

1. Fire the grill to 350F. Use desired wood pellets when cooking. Close the lid and preheat for 15 minutes.
2. Brush the corn with oil and season with salt and pepper to taste.
3. Place the corn on the grill grate and cook for 10 minutes. Make sure to flip the corn halfway through the cooking time for even cooking.
4. Meanwhile, mix the butter and honey in a small bowl. Set aside.
5. Once the corn is cooked, remove it from the grill and brush it with the honey butter sauce.

Nutrition Info: Calories per serving: 387; Protein: 5g; Carbs: 51.2g; Fat: 21.6g Sugar: 28.2g

8. Roasted Parmesan Cheese Broccoli

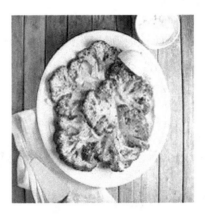

Servings: 3 To 4

Cooking Time: 45 Minutes

Ingredients:

- 3cups broccoli stems trimmed

- 1tbsp lemon juice

- 1tbsp olive oil

- 2garlic cloves, minced

- 1/2 tsp kosher salt

- 1/2 tsp ground black pepper

- 1tsp lemon zest

- 1/8 cup parmesan cheese, grated

Directions:

1. Preheat pellet grill to 375°F.

2. Place broccoli in a resealable bag. Add lemon juice, olive oil, garlic cloves, salt, and pepper. Seal the bag and toss to combine. Let the mixture marinate for 30 minutes.

3. Pour broccoli into a grill basket. Place basket on grill grates to roast. Grill broccoli for 14-18 minutes, flipping broccoli halfway through. Grill until tender yet a little crispy on the outside.

4. Remove broccoli from grill and place on a serving dish – zest with lemon and top with grated parmesan cheese. Serve immediately and enjoy!

Nutrition Info: Calories: 82.6 Fat: 4.6 g Cholesterol: 1.8 mg Carbohydrate: 8.1 g Fiber: 4.6 g Sugar: 0 Protein: 5.5

9. Smoked Mushrooms

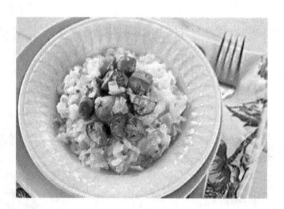

Servings: 2

Cooking Time: 45 Minutes

Ingredients:

- 4 cups whole baby portobello, cleaned

- 1 tbsp canola oil

- 1 tbsp onion powder

- 1 tbsp garlic, granulated

- 1 tbsp salt

- 1 tbsp pepper

Directions:

1. Place all the ingredients in a bowl, mix, and combine.

2. Set yours to 180F.

3. Place the mushrooms on the grill directly and smoke for about 30 minutes.

4. Increase heat to high and cook the mushroom for another 15 minutes.

5. Serve warm and enjoy!

Nutrition Info: Calories 118, Total fat 7.6g, Saturated fat 0.6g, Total carbs 10.8g, Net carbs 8.3g, Protein 5.4g, Sugars 3.7g, Fiber 2.5g, Sodium 3500mg, Potassium 536mg

10. Cajun Style Grilled Corn

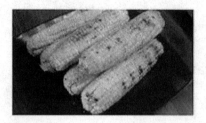

Servings: 4

Cooking Time: 25 Minutes

Ingredients:

- Four ears corn, with husks

- 1tsp dried oregano

- 1tsp paprika

- 1tsp garlic powder

- 1tsp onion powder

- 1/2 tsp kosher salt

- 1/2 tsp ground black pepper

- 1/4 tsp dried thyme

- 1/4 tsp cayenne pepper

- 2tsp butter, melted

Directions:

1. Preheat pellet grill to 375°F.

2. Peel husks back but do not remove. Scrub and remove silks.

3. Mix oregano, paprika, garlic powder, onion powder, salt, pepper, thyme, and cayenne in a small bowl.

4. Brush melted butter over corn.

5. Rub seasoning mixture over each ear of corn. Pull husks up and place corn on grill grates. Grill for about 12-15 minutes, turning occasionally.

6. Remove from grill and allow to cool for about 5 minutes. Remove husks, then serve and enjoy!

Nutrition Info: Calories: 278 Fat: 17.4 g Cholesterol: 40.7 mg Carbohydrate: 30.6 g Fiber: 4.5 g Sugar: 4.6 g Protein: 5.4 g

11. Smoked Baked Beans

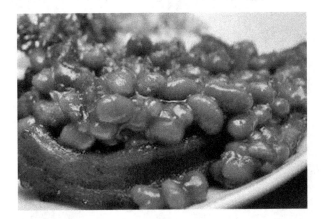

Servings: 12

Cooking Time: 3 Hours

Ingredients:

- 1 medium yellow onion diced

- 3 jalapenos

- 56 oz pork and beans

- 3/4 cup barbeque sauce

- 1/2 cup dark brown sugar

- 1/4 cup apple cider vinegar

- 2 tbsp Dijon mustard

- 2 tbsp molasses

Directions:

1. Preheat, the smoker to 250°F. Pour the beans along with all the liquid in a pan. Add brown sugar, barbeque sauce, Dijon mustard, apple cider vinegar, and molasses. Stir. Place the pan on one of the racks. Smoke for 3 hours until thickened. Remove after 3 hours. Serve

Nutrition Info: Calories: 214 Cal Fat: 2 g Carbohydrates: 42 g   Protein: 7 g Fiber: 7 g

12. Split Pea Soup With Mushrooms

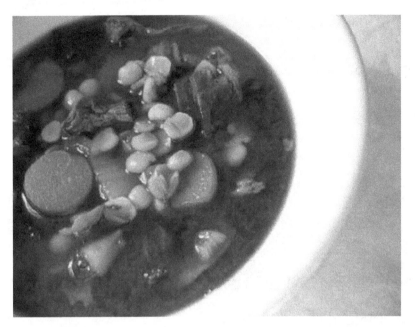

Servings: 4

Cooking Time: 35 Minutes

Ingredients:

- 2tbsp. Olive Oil

- 3Garlic cloves, minced

- 3tbsp. Parsley, fresh and chopped

- 2Carrots chopped

- 1.2/3 cup Green Peas

- 9cups Water

- 2tsp. Salt

- 1/4 tsp. Black Pepper

- 1lb. Portobello Mushrooms

- 1Bay Leaf

- 2Celery Ribs, chopped

- 1Onion quartered

- 1/2 tsp. Thyme, dried

- 6tbsp. Parmesan Cheese, grated

Directions:

1. First, keep oil, onion, and garlic in the blender pitcher.

2. Next, select the 'saute' button.

3. Once sautéed, stir in the rest of the ingredients, excluding parsley and cheese.

4. Then, press the 'hearty soup' button.

5. Finally, transfer the soup among the serving bowls and garnish it with parsley and cheese.

Nutrition Info: Calories: 61 Fat: 1.1 g Total Carbs: 10 g Fiber: 1.9 g Sugar: 3.2 g Protein: 3.2 g Cholesterol: 0

13. Smoked Brussels Sprouts

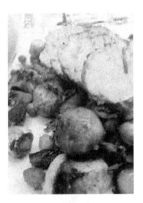

Servings: 6

Cooking Time: 45 Minutes

Ingredients:

- 1-1/2 pounds Brussels sprouts

- Two cloves of garlic minced

- 2 tbsp extra virgin olive oil

- Sea salt and cracked black pepper

Directions:

1. Rinse sprouts

2. Remove the outer leaves and brown bottoms off the sprouts.

3. Place sprouts in a large bowl, then coat with olive oil.

4. Add a coat of garlic, salt, and pepper and transfer them to the pan.

5. Add to the top rack of the smoker with water and woodchips.

6. Smoke for 45 minutes or until it reaches 250°F temperature.

7. Serve

Nutrition Info: Calories: 84 Cal Fat: 4.9 g Carbohydrates: 7.2 g   Protein: 2.6 g Fiber: 2.9 g

14. Roasted Green Beans With Bacon

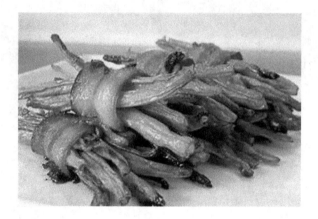

Servings: 6

Cooking Time: 20 Minutes

Ingredients:

- 1-pound green beans

- 4 strips bacon, cut into small pieces

- 4 tablespoons extra virgin olive oil

- 2 cloves garlic, minced

- 1 teaspoon salt

Directions:

1. Fire the grill to 400F. Use desired wood pellets when cooking. Close the lid and preheat for 15 minutes.

2. Toss all ingredients on a sheet tray and spread out evenly.

3. Place the tray on the grill grate and roast for 20 minutes.

Nutrition Info: Calories per serving: 65 ; Protein: 1.3g; Carbs: 3.8g; Fat: 5.3g Sugar: 0.6g

15. Stuffed Grilled Zucchini

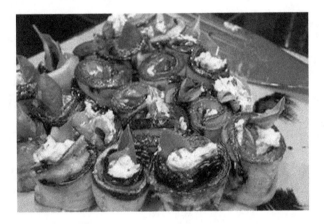

Servings: 4

Cooking Time: 10 Minutes

Ingredients:

*   4 zucchini, medium

*   5 tbsp olive oil, divided

*   2 tbsp red onion, finely chopped

- 1/4 tbsp garlic, minced

- 1/2 cup bread crumbs, dry

- 1/2 cup shredded mozzarella cheese, part-skim

- 1/2 tbsp salt

- 1 tbsp fresh mint, minced

- 3 tbsp parmesan cheese, grated

Directions:

1. Halve zucchini lengthwise and scoop pulp ou. Leave 1/4 -inch shell. Now brush using 2 tbsp oil, set aside, and chop the pulp.

2. Saute onion and pulp in a skillet, large, then add garlic and cook for about 1 minute.

3. Add bread crumbs and cook while stirring for about 2 minutes until golden brown.

4. Remove everything from heat, then stir in mozzarella cheese, salt, and mint. Scoop into the zucchini shells and splash with parmesan cheese.

5. Preheat yours to 375F.

6. Place stuffed zucchini on the grill and grill while covered for about 8-10 minutes until tender.

7. Serve warm and enjoy.

Nutrition Info: Calories 186, Total fat 10g, Saturated fat 3g, Total carbs 17g, Net carbs 14g, Protein 9g, Sugars 4g, Fiber 3g, Sodium 553mg, Potassium 237mg

16. Grilled Zucchini

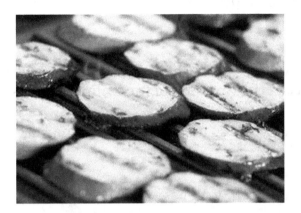

Servings: 6

Cooking Time: 10 Minutes

Ingredients:

- 4 medium zucchini

- 2 tablespoons olive oil

- 1 tablespoon sherry vinegar

- 2 sprigs of thyme, leaves chopped

- ½ teaspoon salt

- 1/3 teaspoon ground black pepper

Directions:

1. Switch on the grill, fill the grill hopper with oak flavored wood pellets, power the grill on by using the control panel, select 'smoke' on the temperature dial, or set the temperature to 350 degrees F and let it preheat for a minimum of 5 minutes.

2. Meanwhile, cut the ends of each zucchini, cut each in half, and then into thirds and place in a plastic bag.

3. Add remaining ingredients, seal the bag, and shake well to coat zucchini pieces.

4. When the grill has preheated, open the lid, place zucchini on the grill grate, shut the grill, and smoke for 4 minutes per side.

5. When done, transfer zucchini to a dish, garnish with more thyme and then serve.

Nutrition Info: Calories: 74 Cal ;Fat: 5.4 g ;Carbs: 6.1 g ;Protein: 2.6 g ;Fiber: 2.3 g

Poultry Recipes

17. Wings

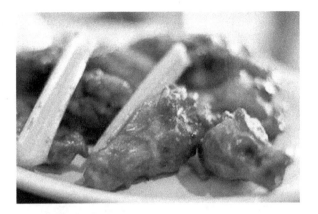

Servings: 4

Cooking Time: 15 Minutes

Ingredients:

- Fresh chicken wings
- Salt to taste
- Pepper to taste
- Garlic powder
- Onion powder
- Cayenne
- Paprika
- Seasoning salt
- Barbeque sauce to taste

Directions:

1. Preheat the wood pellet grill to low. Mix seasoning and coat on chicken. Put the wings on the grill and cook. Place the wings on the grill and cook for 20 minutes or until the wings are fully cooked. Let rest cool for 5 minutes, then toss with barbeque sauce. Serve with orzo and salad. Enjoy.

Nutrition Info: Calories: 311 Cal Fat: 22 g Carbohydrates: 22 g Protein: 22 g Fiber: 3 g

18. Grilled Chicken

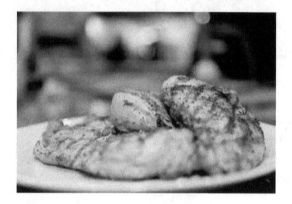

Servings: 6

Cooking Time: 1 Hour 10 Minutes;

Ingredients:

*   5 lb. whole chicken

*   1/2 cup oil

*   chicken rub

Directions:

1. Preheat on the smoke setting with the lid open for 5 minutes. Close the lid and let it heat for 15 minutes or until it reaches 450...

2. Use baker's twine to tie the chicken legs together, then rub it with oil. Coat the chicken with the rub and place it on the grill.

3. Grill for 70 minutes with the lid closed or until it reaches an internal temperature of 165F.

4. Remove the chicken from the and let rest for 15 minutes. Cut and serve.

Nutrition Info: Calories 935, Total fat 53g, Saturated fat 15g, Total carbs 5g, Net carbs 2g Protein 107g, Sugars 0g, Fiber 2g, Sodium 320mg

19. Smoked Turkey Breast

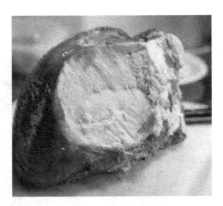

Servings: 2 To 4

Cooking Time: 1 To 2 Hours

Ingredients:

- 1 (3-pound) turkey breast

- Salt

- Freshly ground black pepper

- 1 teaspoon garlic powder

Directions:

1. Supply your smoker with wood pellets and follow the manufacturer's specific start-up procedure. Preheat the grill, with the lid closed, to 180°F.

2. Season the turkey breast all over with salt, pepper, and garlic powder.

3. Place the breast directly on the grill grate and smoke for 1 hour.

4. Increase the grill's temperature to 350°F and continue to cook until the turkey's internal temperature reaches 170°F. Remove the breast from the grill and serve immediately.

20. Mini Turducken Roulade

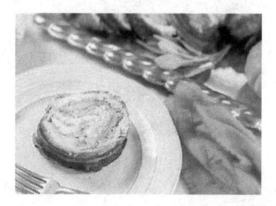

Servings: 6

Cooking Time: 2 Hours

Ingredients:

- 1 (16-ounce) boneless turkey breast

- 1 (8-to 10-ounce) boneless duck breast

- 1 (8-ounce) boneless, skinless chicken breast

- Salt

- Freshly ground black pepper

- 2 cups Italian dressing

- 2 tablespoons Cajun seasoning

- 1 cup prepared seasoned stuffing mix

- 8 slices bacon

- Butcher's string

Directions:

1. Butterfly the turkey, duck, and chicken breasts, cover with plastic wrap, and, using a mallet, flatten each ½ inch thick.

2. Season all the meat on both sides with a little salt and pepper.

3. In a medium bowl, combine the Italian dressing and Cajun seasoning. Spread one-fourth of the mixture on top of the flattened turkey breast.

4. Place the duck breast on top of the turkey, spread it with one-fourth of the dressing mixture, and top with the stuffing mix.

5. Place the chicken breast on top of the duck and spread with one-fourth of the dressing mixture.

6. Supply your smoker with wood pellets and follow the manufacturer's specific start-up procedure. Preheat, with the lid, closed to 275°F.

7. Tightly roll up the stack, tie with butcher's string, and slather the whole thing with the remaining dressing mixture.

8. Wrap the bacon slices around the turducken and secure with toothpicks, or try making a bacon weave (see the technique for this in the Jalapeño-Bacon Pork Tenderloin recipe).

9. Place the turducken roulade in a roasting pan. Transfer to the grill, close the lid, and roast for 2 hours, or until a meat thermometer inserted in the turducken reads 165°F. Tent with aluminum foil in the last 30 minutes, if necessary, to keep from over-browning.

10.   Let the turducken rest for 15 to 20 minutes before carving. Serve warm.

21. Herb Roasted Turkey

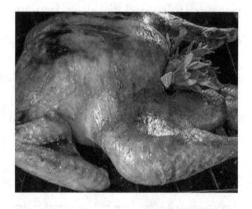

Servings: 12

Cooking Time: 3 Hours And 30 Minutes

Ingredients:

- 14 pounds turkey, cleaned

- Two tablespoons chopped mixed herbs

- Pork and poultry rub as needed

- 1/4 teaspoon ground black pepper

- Three tablespoons butter, unsalted, melted

- Eight tablespoons butter, unsalted, softened

- 2 cups chicken broth

Directions:

1. Clean the turkey by removing the giblets, wash it inside out, pat dry with paper towels, then place it on a roasting pan and tuck the turkey wings by tiring with butcher's string.

2. Switch on the grill, fill the grill hopper with hickory flavored wood pellets, power the grill on by using the control panel, select 'smoke' on the temperature dial, or set the temperature to 325 degrees F and let it preheat for a minimum of 15 minutes.

3. Meanwhile, prepare herb butter, take a small bowl, place the softened butter in it, add black pepper and mixed herbs, and beat until fluffy.

4. Place some of the prepared herb butter underneath the turkey's skin by using a wooden spoon handle and massage the skin to distribute butter evenly.

5. Then rub the exterior of the turkey with melted butter, season with pork and poultry rub, and pour the broth in the roasting pan.

6. When the grill has preheated, open the lid, place the roasting pan containing turkey on the grill grate, shut the grill, and smoke for 3 hours and 30 minutes until the internal temperature reaches 165 degrees F and the top has turned golden brown.

7. When done, transfer turkey to a cutting board, let it rest for 30 minutes, then carve it into slices and serve.

Nutrition Info: Calories: 154.6 Cal ;Fat: 3.1 g ;Carbs: 8.4 g ;Protein: 28.8 g ;Fiber: 0.4 g

22. Lemon Chicken Breast

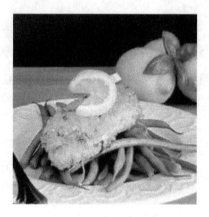

Servings: 4

Cooking Time: 30 Minutes

Ingredients:

- 6 chicken breasts, skinless and boneless

- ½ cup oil

- 1-3 fresh thyme sprigs

- 1teaspoon ground black pepper

- 2teaspoon salt

- 2teaspoons honey

- 1garlic clove, chopped

- 1lemon, juiced and zested

- Lemon wedges

Directions:

1. Take a bowl and prepare the marinade by mixing thyme, pepper, salt, honey, garlic, lemon zest, and juice. Mix well until dissolved

2. Add oil and whisk

3. Clean breasts and pat them dry, place in a bag alongside marinade, and let them sit in the fridge for 4 hours

4. Preheat your smoker to 400 degrees F

5. Drain chicken and smoke until the internal temperature reaches 165 degrees, for about 15 minutes

6. Serve and enjoy!

Nutrition Info: Calories: 230 Fats: 7g Carbs: 1g Fiber: 2g

23. Applewood-smoked Whole Turkey

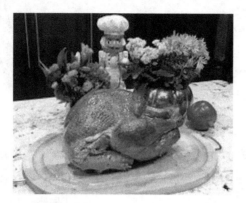

Servings: 6 To 8

Cooking Time: 5 To 6 Hours

Ingredients:

- 1 (10- to 12-pound) turkey, giblets removed

- Extra-virgin olive oil, for rubbing

- ¼ cup poultry seasoning

- 8 tablespoons (1 stick) unsalted butter, melted

- ½ cup apple juice

- 2 teaspoons dried sage

- 2 teaspoons dried thyme

Directions:

1. Supply your smoker with wood pellets and follow the manufacturer's specific start-up procedure. Preheat, with the lid, closed to 250°F.

2. Rub the turkey with oil and season with the poultry seasoning inside and out, getting under the skin.

3. In a bowl, combine the melted butter, apple juice, sage, and thyme to basting.

4. Put the turkey in a roasting pan, place on the grill, close the lid, and grill for 5 to 6 hours, basting every hour until the skin is brown and crispy, or until a meat thermometer inserted in the thickest part of the thigh reads 165°F.

5. Let the bird rest for 15 to 20 minutes before carving.

24. Spatchcocked Turkey

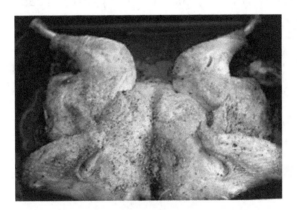

Servings: 10 To 14

Cooking Time: 2 Hours

Ingredients:

- 1 whole turkey

- 2 tablespoons olive oil

- 1 batch Chicken Rub

Directions:

1. Supply your smoker with wood pellets and follow the manufacturer's specific start-up procedure. Preheat the grill, with the lid closed, to 350°F.

2. To remove the turkey's backbone, place the turkey on a work surface, on its breast. Using kitchen shears, cut along one side of the turkey's backbone and then the other. Pull out the bone.

3. Once the backbone is removed, turn the turkey breast-side up and flatten it.

4. Coat the turkey with olive oil and season it on both sides with the rub. Using your hands, work the rub into the meat and skin.

5. Place the turkey directly on the grill grate, breast-side up, and cook until its internal temperature reaches 170°F.

6. Remove the turkey from the grill and let it rest for 10 minutes before carving and serving.

25. Garlic Parmesan Chicken Wings

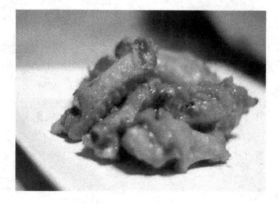

Servings: 6

Cooking Time: 20 Minutes

Ingredients:

- 5 pounds of chicken wings

- 1/2 cup chicken rub

- 3 tablespoons chopped parsley

- 1 cup shredded parmesan cheese

- For the Sauce:

- 5 teaspoons minced garlic

- 2 tablespoons chicken rub

- 1 cup butter, unsalted

Directions:

1. Switch on the grill, fill the grill hopper with cherry flavored wood pellets, power the grill on by using the control panel, select 'smoke' on the temperature dial, or set the temperature to 450 degrees F and let it preheat for a minimum of 15 minutes.

2. Meanwhile, take a large bowl, place chicken wings in it, sprinkle with chicken rub, and toss until well coated.

3. When the grill has preheated, open the lid, place chicken wings on the grill grate, shut the grill, and smoke for 10 minutes per side until the internal temperature reaches 165 degrees F.

4. Meanwhile, prepare the sauce and for this, take a medium saucepan, place it over medium heat, add all the ingredients for the sauce in it and cook for 10 minutes until smooth, set aside until required.

5.   When done, transfer chicken wings to a dish, top with prepared sauce, toss until mixed, garnish with cheese and parsley and then serve.

Nutrition Info: Calories: 180 Cal ;Fat: 1 g ;Carbs: 8 g ;Protein: 0 g ;Fiber: 0 g

26. Trager Smoked Spatchcock Turkey

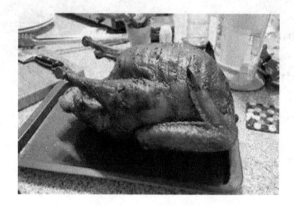

Servings: 8

Cooking Time: 1 Hour 15 Minutes;

Ingredients:

- 1 turkey

- 1/2 cup melted butter

- 1/4 cup chicken rub

- 1 tbsp onion powder

- 1 tbsp garlic powder

- 1 tbsp rubbed sage

Directions:

1. Preheat your to high temperature.

2. Place the turkey on a chopping board with the breast side down and the legs pointing towards you.

3. Cut either side of the turkey backbone to remove the spine. Flip the turkey and place it on a pan

4. Season both sides with the seasonings and place it on the grill skin side up on the grill.

5. Cook for 30 minutes, reduce temperature, and cook for 45 more minutes or until the internal temperature reaches 165F.

6. Remove from the and let rest for 15 minutes before slicing and serving.

Nutrition Info: Calories 156, Total fat 16g, Saturated fat 2g, Total carbs 1g, Net carbs 1g Protein 2g, Sugars 2g, Fiber 5g, Sodium 19mg

27. Grilled Buffalo Chicken Legs

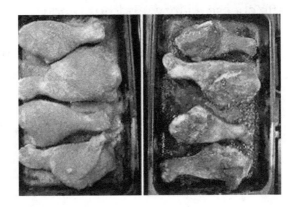

Servings: 8

Cooking Time: 1 Hour 15 Minutes;

Ingredients:

- 12 chicken legs

- 1/2 tbsp salt

- 1 tbsp buffalo seasoning

- 1 cup Buffalo sauce

Directions:

1. Preheat your to 325F.

2. Toss the chicken legs in salt and seasoning, then place them on the preheated grill.

3. Grill for 40 minutes, turning twice through the cooking.

4. Increase the heat and cook for ten more minutes. Brush the chicken legs and brush with buffalo sauce. Cook for an additional 10 minutes or until the internal temperature reaches 165F.

5. Remove from the and brush with more buffalo sauce.

6. Serve with blue cheese, celery, and hot ranch.

Nutrition Info: Calories 956, Total fat 47g, Saturated fat 13g, Total carbs 1g, Net carbs 1g Protein 124g, Sugars 0g, Fiber 0g, Sodium 1750mg

Beef, Pork & Lamb Recipes

28. County Ribs

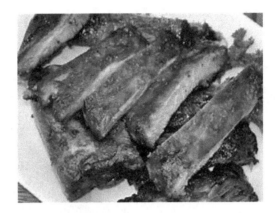

Preparation Time: 15 Minutes

Cooking Time: 3 Hours

Servings: 4

Ingredients:

- 4 pounds country-style ribs

- Pork ribs to taste.

- 2 cups apple juice

- ½ stick butter, melted.

- 18 ounces BBQ sauce

Directions:

1. Take your drip pan and add water. Cover with aluminum foil.

2. Pre-heat your smoker to 275 degrees F

3. Season country style ribs from all sides

4. Use water fill water pan halfway through and place it over drip pan.

5. Add wood chips to the side tray.

6. Transfer the ribs to your smoker and smoke for 1 hour and 15 minutes until the internal temperature reaches 160 degrees F.

7. Take foil pan and mix melted butter, apple juice, 15 ounces BBQ sauce and put ribs back in the pan, cover with foil.

8. Transfer back to smoker and smoke for 1 hour 15 minutes more until the internal temperature reaches 195 degrees F.

9. Take ribs out from liquid, place them on racks, glaze ribs with more BBQ sauce, and smoke for 10 minutes more.

10. Take them out and let them rest for 10 minutes, serve, and enjoy!

Nutrition:

Calories: 251

Fat: 25g

Carbohydrates: 35g

Protein: 76g

29. Wow-Pork Tenderloin

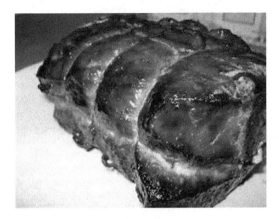

Preparation Time: 15 Minutes

Cooking Time: 3 Hours

Servings: 4

Ingredients:

- One pork tenderloin

- ¼ cup BBQ sauce

- Three tablespoons dry rub

Directions:

1. Take your drip pan and add water. Cover with aluminum foil.

2. Pre-heat your smoker to 225 degrees F

3. Rub the spice blend all finished the pork tenderloin.

4. Use water fill water pan halfway through and place it over drip pan.

5. Add wood chips to the side tray.

6. Transfer pork meat to your smoker and smoke for 3 hours until the internal temperature reaches 145 degrees F.

7. Brush the BBQ sauce over pork and let it rest.

8. Serve and enjoy!

Nutrition:

Calories: 405

Fat: 9g

Carbohydrates: 15g

Protein: 59g

30. Awesome Pork Shoulder

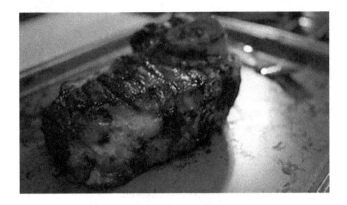

Preparation Time: 15 Minutes + 24 Hours

Cooking Time: 12 Hours

Servings: 4

Ingredients:

- 8 pounds of pork shoulder

For Rub

- One teaspoon dry mustard

- One teaspoon black pepper

- One teaspoon cumin

- One teaspoon oregano

- One teaspoon cayenne pepper

- 1/3 cup salt

- ¼ cup garlic powder

- ½ cup paprika

- 1/3 cup brown sugar

- 2/3 cup sugar

Directions:

1. Bring your pork under salted water for 18 hours.

2. Pull the pork out from the brine and let it sit for 1 hour.

3. Rub mustard all over the pork.

4. Take a bowl and mix all rub ingredients. Rub mixture all over the meat.

5. Wrap meat and leave it overnight.

6. Take your drip pan and add water. Cover with aluminum foil. Pre-heat your smoker to 250 degrees F

7. Use water fill water pan halfway through and place it over drip pan. Add wood chips to the side tray.

8. Transfer meat to smoker and smoke for 6 hours

9. Take the pork out and wrap in foil, smoke for 6 hours more at 195 degrees F.

10. Shred and serve.

11. Enjoy!

Nutrition:

Calories: 965

Fat: 65g

Carbohydrates: 19g

Protein: 71g

31. Premium Sausage Hash

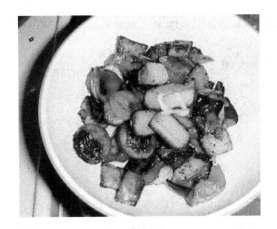

Preparation Time: 30 Minutes

Cooking Time: 45 Minutes

Servings: 4

Ingredients:

- Nonstick cooking spray

- Two finely minced garlic cloves

- One teaspoon basil, dried

- One teaspoon oregano, dried

- One teaspoon onion powder

- One teaspoon of salt

- 4-6 cooked smoker Italian Sausage (Sliced)

- One large-sized bell pepper, diced.

- One large onion, diced.

- Three potatoes cut into 1-inch cubes.

- Three tablespoons of olive oil

- French bread for serving.

Directions:

1. Pre-heat your smoker to 225 degrees Fahrenheit using your desired wood chips.

2. Cover the smoker grill rack with foil and coat with cooking spray.

3. Take a small bowl and add garlic, oregano, basil, onion powder, and season the mix with salt and pepper.

4. Take a large bowl and add sausage slices, bell pepper, potatoes, onion, olive oil, and spice mix.

5. Mix well and spread the mixture on your foil-covered rack.

6. Place the rack in your smoker and smoke for 45 minutes.

7. Serve with your French bread.

8. Enjoy!

Nutrition:

Calories: 193

Fats: 10g

Carbs: 15g

Fiber: 2g

32. Explosive Smoky Bacon

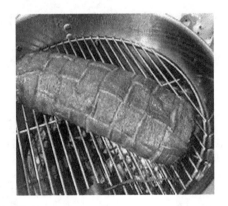

Preparation Time: 20 Minutes

Cooking Time: 2 Hours and 10 Minutes

Servings: 10

Ingredients:

- 1-pound thick-cut bacon

- One tablespoon BBQ spice rub

- 2 pounds bulk pork sausage

- One cup cheddar cheese, shredded.

- Four garlic cloves, minced.

- 18 ounces BBQ sauce

Directions:

1. Take your drip pan and add water. Cover with aluminum foil.

2. Pre-heat your smoker to 225 degrees F

3. Use water fill water pan halfway through and place it over drip pan.

4. Add wood chips to the side tray.

5. Reserve about ½ a pound of your bacon for cooking later

6. Lay 2 strips of your remaining bacon on a clean surface in an X formation.

7. Alternate the horizontal and vertical bacon strips by waving them tightly in an over and under to create a lattice-like pattern.

8. Sprinkle one teaspoon of BBQ rub over the woven bacon

9. Arrange ½ a pound of your bacon in a large-sized skillet and cook them for 10 minutes over medium-high heat.

10. Drain the cooked slices on a kitchen towel and crumble them.

11. Place your sausages in a large-sized re-sealable bag.

12. While the sausages are still in the bag, roll them out to a square with the same size as the woven bacon.

13. Cut off the bag from the sausage and arrange the sausage over the woven bacon.

14. Toss away the bag.

15. Sprinkle some crumbled bacon, green onions, cheddar cheese, and garlic over the rolled sausages.

16. Pour about ¾ bottle of your BBQ sauce over the sausage and season with some more BBQ rub.

17. Roll up the woven bacon tightly all around the sausage, forming a loaf.

18. Cook the bacon-sausage loaf in your smoker for about one and a ½ hours.

19. Brush up the woven bacon with the remaining BBQ sauce and keep smoking for about 30 minutes until the center of the loaf is no longer pink.

20. Use an instant thermometer to check if the internal temperature is at least 165 degrees Fahrenheit.

21. If yes, then take it out and let it rest for 30 minutes.

22. Slice and serve!

Nutrition:

Calories: 507

Fats: 36g

Carbs: 20g

Fiber: 2g

33. Grilled Lamb Burgers

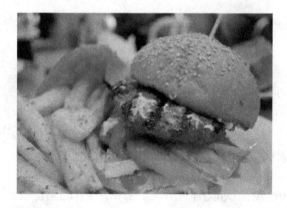

Preparation Time: 10 minutes

Cooking Time: 15 minutes

Servings: 5

Ingredients:

- 1 1/4 pounds of ground lamb.

- One egg.

- One teaspoon of dried oregano.

- One teaspoon of dry sherry.

- One teaspoon of white wine vinegar.

- Four minced cloves of garlic.

- Red pepper

- 1/2 cup of chopped green onions.

- One tablespoon of chopped mint.

- Two tablespoons of chopped cilantro.

- Two tablespoons of dry breadcrumbs.

- 1/8 teaspoon of salt to taste.

- 1/4 teaspoon of ground black pepper to taste.

- Five hamburger buns.

Directions:

1. Preheat a Wood Pellet Smoker or Grill to 350-450 degrees F, then grease it grates.

2. Using a large mixing bowl, add all the ingredients on the list aside from the buns, then mix properly to combine with clean hands.

3. Make about five patties out of the mixture, then set aside.

4. Place the lamb patties on the preheated grill and cook for about seven to nine minutes, turning only once until an inserted thermometer reads 160 degrees F.

5. Serve the lamb burgers on the hamburger, add your favorite toppings, and enjoy.

Nutrition:

Calories: 376 Cal

Fat: 18.5 g

Carbohydrates: 25.4 g

Protein: 25.5 g

Fiber: 1.6 g

34. Lamb Chops

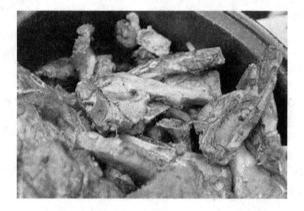

Preparation Time: 10 minutes

Cooking Time: 12 minutes

Servings: 6

Ingredients:

- 6 (6-ounce) lamb chops

- 3 tablespoons olive oil

- Ground black pepper

Directions:

1. Preheat the pallet grill to 450 degrees F.

2. Coat the lamb chops with oil and then season with salt and black pepper evenly.

3. Arrange the chops in a pallet grill grate and cook for about 4-6 minutes per side.

Nutrition:

Calories: 376 Cal

Fat: 19.5 g

Carbohydrates: 0 g

Protein: 47.8 g

Fiber: 0 g

35. Lamb Ribs Rack

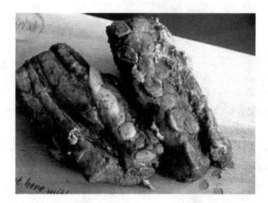

Preparation Time: 10 minutes

Cooking Time: 2 hours

Servings: 2

Ingredients:

- Two tablespoons fresh sage

- Two tablespoons fresh rosemary

- Two tablespoons fresh thyme

- Two peeled garlic cloves

- One tablespoon honey

- Black pepper

- ¼ cup olive oil

- 1 (1½-pound) trimmed rack lamb ribs.

Directions:

1. Combine all ingredients.

2. While the motor is running, slowly add oil and pulse till a smooth paste is formed.

3. Coat the rib rack with paste generously and refrigerate for about 2 hours.

4. Preheat the pallet grill to 225 degrees F.

5. Arrange the rib rack in pallet grill and cook for about 2 hours.

6. Remove the rib rack from the pallet grill and transfer onto a cutting board for about 10-15 minutes before slicing.

7. With a sharp knife, cut the rib rack into equal-sized individual ribs and serve.

Nutrition:

Calories: 826 Cal

Fat: 44.1 g

Carbohydrates: 5.4 g

Protein: 96.3 g

Fiber: 1 g

36. Leg of a Lamb

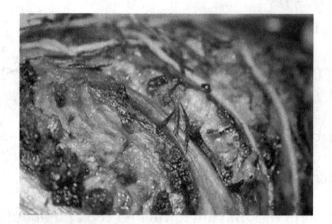

Preparation Time: 10 minutes

Cooking Time: 2 hours and 30 minutes

Servings: 10

Ingredients:

- 1 (8-ounce) package softened cream cheese.

- ¼ cup cooked and crumbled bacon.

- One seeded and chopped jalapeño pepper.

- One tablespoon crushed dried rosemary.

- Two teaspoons garlic powder

- One teaspoon onion powder

- One teaspoon paprika

- One teaspoon cayenne pepper

- Salt, to taste

- 1 (4-5-pound) butterflied leg of lamb

- 2-3 tablespoons olive oil

Directions:

1. For filling in a bowl, add all ingredients and mix till well combined.

2. For spice mixture in another small bowl, mix all ingredients.

3. Place the leg of lamb onto a smooth surface. Sprinkle the inside of the leg with some spice mixture.

4. Place filling mixture over the inside surface evenly. Roll the leg of lamb tightly, and with a butcher's twine, tie the roll to secure the filling.

5. Coat the outer side of the roll with olive oil evenly, and then sprinkle with spice mixture.

6. Preheat the pallet grill to 225-240 degrees F.

7. Arrange the leg of lamb in a pallet grill and cook for about 2-2½ hours. Remove the leg of lamb from the pallet grill and transfer it onto a cutting board.

8. With a piece of foil, cover the leg loosely and transfer onto a cutting board for about 20-25 minutes before slicing.

9. With a sharp knife, cut the leg of lamb in desired sized slices and serve.

Nutrition:

Calories: 715 Cal

Fat: 38.9 g

Carbohydrates: 2.2 g

Protein: 84.6 g

Fiber: 0.1 g

37. Lamb Breast

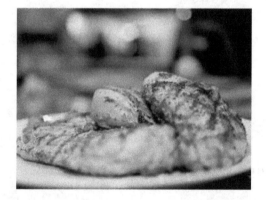

Preparation Time: 10 minutes

Cooking Time: 2 hours and 40 minutes

Servings: 2

Ingredients:

- 1 (2-pound) trimmed bone-in lamb breast.

- ½ cup white vinegar

- ¼ cup yellow mustard

- ½ cup BBQ rub

Directions:

1. Preheat the pallet grill to 225 degrees F.

2. Rinse the lamb breast with vinegar evenly.

3. Coat lamb breast with mustard and season with BBQ rub evenly.

4. Arrange lamb breast in pallet grill and cook for about 2-2½ hours.

5. Remove the lamb breast from the pallet grill and transfer onto a cutting board for about 10 minutes before slicing.

6. With a sharp knife, cut the lamb breast in desired-sized slices and serve.

Nutrition:

Calories: 877 Cal

Fat: 34.5 g

Carbohydrates: 2.2 g

Protein: 128.7 g

Fiber: 0 g

38. New York Strip

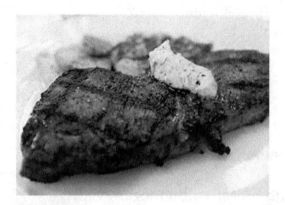

Servings: 6

Cooking Time: 15 Minutes

Ingredients:

- 3 New York strips

- Salt and pepper

Directions:

1. If the steak is in the fridge, remove it 30 minutes before cooking.

2. Preheat the

3. to 450F.

4. Meanwhile, season the steak generously with salt and pepper. Place it on the grill and let it cook for 5 minutes per side or until the internal temperature reaches 1280F.

5. Rest for 10 minutes.

Nutrition Info: Calories: 198 Cal Fat: 14 g Carbohydrates: 0 g   Protein: 17 g Fiber: 0 g

39. Lamb Shank

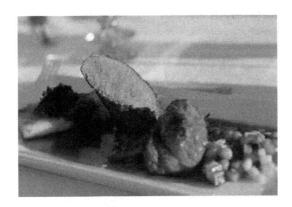

Servings: 6

Cooking Time: 4 Hours

Ingredients:

- 8-ounce red wine

- 2-ounce whiskey

- 2 tablespoons minced fresh rosemary

- 1 tablespoon minced garlic

- Black pepper

- 6 (1¼-pound) lamb shanks

Directions:

1. In a bowl, add all ingredients except lamb shank and mix till well combined.

2. In a large resealable bag, add marinade and lamb shank.

3. Seal the bag and shake to coat completely.

4. Refrigerate for about 24 hours.

5. Preheat the pallet grill to 225 degrees F.

6. Arrange the leg of lamb in a pallet grill and cook for about 4 hours.

Nutrition Info: Calories: 1507 Cal Fat: 62 g Carbohydrates: 68.7 g   Protein:163.3 g Fiber: 6 g

40. Spicy Pork Chops

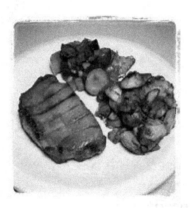

Servings: 4

Cooking Time: 10-15 Minutes

Ingredients:

- 1 tbsp. olive oil

- 2 cloves garlic, crushed and minced

- 1 tbsp. cayenne pepper

- ½ tsp. hot sauce

- ¼ cup lime juice

- 2 tsp. ground cumin

- 1 tsp. ground cinnamon

- 4 pork chops

- Lettuce

Directions:

1. Mix the olive oil, garlic, cayenne pepper, hot sauce, lime juice, cumin, and cinnamon.

2. Pour the mixture into a re-sealable plastic bag. Place the pork chops inside. Seal and turn to coat evenly. Chill in the refrigerator for 4 hours. Grill for 10 to 15 minutes, flipping occasionally.

Nutrition Info: Calories: 196 Cal Fat: 9 g Carbohydrates: 3 g   Protein: 25 g Fiber: 1 g

41. Apple-smoked Bacon

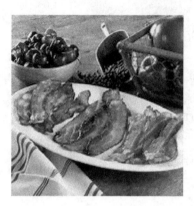

Servings: 4 To 6

Cooking Time: 20 To 30 Minutes

Ingredients:

- 1 (1-pound) package thick-sliced bacon

Directions:

1. Supply your smoker with wood pellets and follow the manufacturer's specific start-up procedure. Preheat the grill, with the lid closed, to 275°F.

2. Supply your smoker with wood pellets and follow the manufacturer's specific start-up procedure. Preheat the grill, with the lid closed, to 275°F.

42. Deliciously Spicy Rack Of Lamb

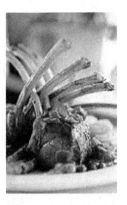

Servings: 6

Cooking Time: 3 Hours

Ingredients:

- 2 tbsp. paprika

- ½ tbsp. coriander seeds

- 1 tsp. cumin seeds

- 1 tsp. ground allspice

- 1 tsp. lemon peel powder

- Salt and freshly ground black pepper, to taste

- 2 (1½-lb.) rack of lamb ribs, trimmed

Directions:

1. Set the Grill temperature to 225 degrees F and preheat with a closed lid for 15 minutes.

2. In a coffee grinder, add all ingredients except rib racks and grind them into a powder.

3. Coat the rib racks with spice mixture generously.

4. Arrange the rib racks onto the grill and cook for about 3 hours.

5. Remove the rib racks from the grill and place them onto a cutting board for about 10-15 minutes before slicing.

6. With a sharp knife, cut the rib racks into equal-sized individual ribs and serve.

Nutrition Info: Calories per serving: 545; Carbohydrates: 1.7g; Protein: 64.4g; Fat: 29.7g; Sugar: 0.3g; Sodium: 221mg; Fiber: 1g

43. Grilled Butter Basted Rib-eye

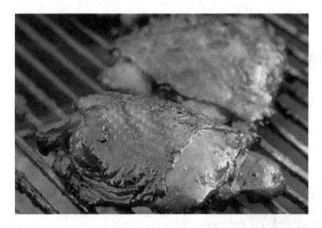

Servings: 4

Cooking Time: 20 Minutes

Ingredients:

- 2 rib-eye steaks, bone-in

- Slat to taste

- Pepper to taste

- 4 tbsp butter, unsalted

Directions:

1. Mix steak, salt, and pepper in a ziplock bag. Seal the bag and mix until the beef is well coated. Ensure you get as much air as possible from the ziplock bag.

2. Set the wood pellet grill temperature to high with a closed lid for 15 minutes. Place a cast iron into the grill.

3. Place the steaks on the hottest spot of the grill and cook for 5 minutes with the lid closed.

4. Open the lid and add butter to the skillet when it's almost melted. Place the steak on the skillet with the grilled side up.

5. Cook for 5 minutes while busting the meat with butter. Close the lid and cook until the internal temperature is 130°F.

6. Remove the steak from the skillet and let rest for 10 minutes before enjoying with the reserved butter.

Nutrition Info: Calories 745, Total fat 65g, Saturated fat 32g, Total Carbs 5g, Net Carbs 5g, Protein 35g, Sugar 0g, Fiber 0g

44. Pork Belly Burnt Ends

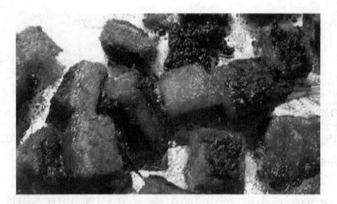

Servings: 8 To 10

Cooking Time: 6 Hours

Ingredients:

- 1 (3-pound) skinless pork belly (if not already skinned, use a sharp boning knife to remove the skin from the belly), cut into 1½- to 2-inch cubes

- One batch Sweet Brown Sugar Rub

- ½ cup honey

- 1 cup The Ultimate BBQ Sauce

- Two tablespoons light brown sugar

Directions:

1. Supply your smoker with wood pellets and follow the manufacturer's specific start-up procedure. Preheat the grill, with the lid closed, to 250°F.

2. Generously season the pork belly cubes with the rub. Using your hands, work the rub into the meat.

3. Place the pork cubes directly on the grill grate and smoke until their internal temperature reaches 195°F.

4. Transfer the cubes from the grill to an aluminum pan. Add the honey, barbecue sauce, and brown sugar. Stir to combine and coat the pork.

5. Place the pan in the grill and smoke the pork for 1 hour, uncovered. Remove the pork from the grill and serve immediately.

45. Simple Grilled Lamb Chops

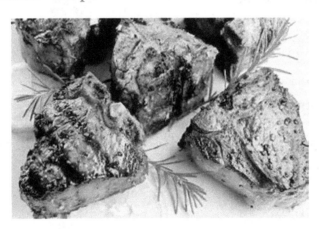

Servings: 6

Cooking Time: 6 Minutes

Ingredients:

- 1/4 cup distilled white vinegar

- 2 tbsp salt

- 1/2 tbsp black pepper

- 1 tbsp garlic, minced

- 1 onion, thinly sliced

- 2 tbsp olive oil

- 2lb lamb chops

Directions:

1. In a resealable bag, mix vinegar, salt, black pepper, garlic, sliced onion, and oil until all salt has dissolved.

2. Add the lamb chops and toss until well coated. Place in the fridge to marinate for 2 hours.

3. Preheat the wood pellet grill to high heat.

4. Remove the lamb from the fridge and discard the marinade. Wrap any exposed bones with foil.

5. Grill the lamb for 3 minutes per side. You can also broil in a broiler for more crispness.

6. Serve and enjoy

Nutrition Info: Calories 519, Total fat 44.8g, Saturated fat 18g, Total Carbs 2.3g, Net Carbs 1.9g, Protein 25g, Sugar1g, Fiber 0.4g, Sodium: 861mg, Potassium 359mg

46. Smoked Sausages

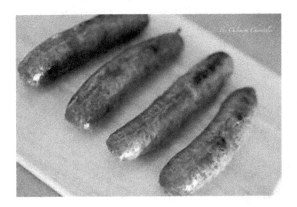

Servings: 4

Cooking Time: 3 Hours

Ingredients:

- 3 pounds ground pork

- 1 tablespoon onion powder

- 1 tablespoon garlic powder

- 1 teaspoon curing salt

- 4 teaspoon black pepper

- 1/2 tablespoon salt

- 1/2 tablespoon ground mustard

- Hog casings, soaked

- 1/2 cup ice water

Directions:

1. Switch on the grill, fill the grill hopper with flavored wood pellets, power the grill on by using the control panel, select 'smoke' on the temperature dial, or set the temperature to 225 degrees F and let it it preheat for a minimum of 15 minutes.

2. Meanwhile, take a medium bowl, place all the ingredients in it except for water and hog casings, and stir until well mixed.

3. Pour in water, stir until incorporated, place the mixture in a sausage stuffer, then stuff the hog casings and tie the link to the desired length.

4. When the grill has preheated, open the lid, place the sausage links on the grill grate, shut the grill, and smoke for 2 to 3 hours until the internal temperature reaches 155 degrees F.

5. When done, transfer sausages to a dish, let them rest for 5 minutes, then slice and serve.

Nutrition Info: Calories: 230 Cal ;Fat: 22 g ;Carbs: 2 g ;Protein: 14 g ;Fiber: 0 g

47. Wood Pellet Smoked Beef Jerky

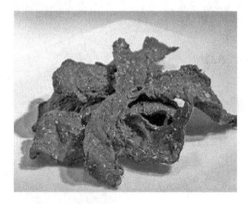

Servings: 10

Cooking Time: 5 Hours

Ingredients:

- 3 lb sirloin steaks, sliced into 1/4 inch thickness

- 2 cups soy sauce

- 1/2 cup brown sugar

- 1 cup pineapple juice

- 2 tbsp sriracha

- 2 tbsp red pepper flake

- 2 tbsp hoisin

- 2 tbsp onion powder

- 2 tbsp rice wine vinegar

- 2 tbsp garlic, minced

Directions:

1. Mix all the ingredients in a ziplock bag. Seal the bag and mix until the beef is well coated. Ensure you get as much air as possible from the ziplock bag.

2. Put the bag in the fridge overnight to let it marinate. Remove the bag from the fridge for 1 hour prior to cooking.

3. Startup your wood pallet grill and set it to a smoke setting. Layout the meat on the grill with half-inch space between them.

4. Let them cook for 5 hours while turning after every 2-1/2 hours.

5. Transfer from the grill and let cool for 30 minutes before serving.

6. Enjoy.

Nutrition Info: Calories 80, Total fat 1g, Saturated fat 0g, Total carbs 5g, Net carbs 5g, Protein 14g, Sugar 5g, Fiber 0g, Sodium: 650mg

48. Bbq Brisket

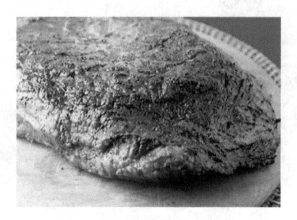

Servings: 8

Cooking Time: 10 Hours

Ingredients:

- 1 beef brisket, about 12 pounds

- Beef rub as needed

Directions:

1. Season beef brisket with beef rub until well coated, place it in a large plastic bag, seal it and let it marinate for a minimum of 12 hours in the refrigerator.

2. When ready to cook, switch on the grill, fill the grill hopper with hickory flavored wood pellets, power the grill on by using the control panel, select 'smoke' on the temperature dial, or set the temperature to 225 degrees F and let it preheat for a minimum of 15 minutes.

3.   When the grill has preheated, open the lid, place marinated brisket on the grill grate fat-side down, shut the grill, and smoke for 6 hours until the internal temperature reaches 160 degrees F.

4.   Then wrap the brisket in foil, return it to the grill grate and cook for 4 hours until the internal temperature reaches 204 degrees F.

5.   When done, transfer brisket to a cutting board, let it rest for 30 minutes, then cut it into slices and serve.

Nutrition Info: Calories: 328 Cal ;Fat: 21 g ;Carbs: 0 g ;Protein: 32 g ;Fiber: - g

49. Bacon Stuffed Smoked Pork Loin

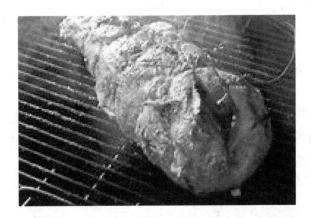

Servings: 4 To 6

Cooking Time: 1 Hour

Ingredients:

- 3 Pound Pork Loin, Butterflied

- As Needed Pork Rub

- 1/4 Cup Walnuts, Chopped

- 1/3 Cup Craisins

- 1 Tablespoon Oregano, fresh

- 1 Tablespoon fresh thyme

- 6 Pieces Asparagus, fresh

- 6 Slices Bacon, sliced

- 1/3 Cup Parmesan cheese, grated

- As Needed Bacon Grease

Directions:

1. Lay down two large pieces of butcher's twine on your work surface. Place butterflied pork loin perpendicular to twine.

2. Season the inside of the pork loin with the pork rub.

3. On one end of the loin, layer in a line all of the ingredients, beginning with the chopped walnuts, craisins, oregano, thyme, and asparagus.

4. Add bacon and top with the parmesan cheese.

5. Starting at the end with all of the fillings, carefully roll up the pork loin and secure on both ends with butcher's twine.

6. Roll the pork loin in the reserved bacon grease and season the outside with more Pork Rub.

7. When ready to cook, set temperature to 180°F and preheat, lid closed for 15 minutes. Place stuffed pork loin directly on the grill grate and smoke for 1 hour.

8. Remove the pork loin; increase the temperature to 350°F and allow to preheat.

9. Place the loin back on the and grill for approximately 30 to 45 minutes or until the temperature reads 135°F on an instant-read thermometer.

10. Move the pork loin to a plate and tent it with aluminum foil. Let it rest for 15 minutes before slicing and serving. Enjoy!

50. Smoked Beef Ribs

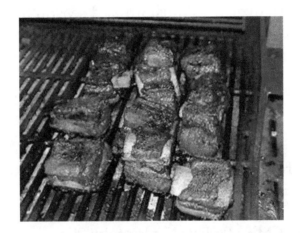

Preparation Time: 25 minutes

Cooking Time: 4 to 6 hours

Servings: 4 to 8

Ingredients:

- 2 (2- or 3-pound) racks beef ribs

- Two tablespoons yellow mustard

- One batch Sweet and Spicy Cinnamon Rub

Directions:

1. Supply your smoker with wood pellets and follow the manufacturer's specific start-up procedure. Allow your griller to preheat with the lid closed to 225°F.

2. Take off the membrane from the backside of the ribs. This can be done by cutting just through the membrane in an X pattern and working a paper towel between the membrane and the ribs to pull it off.

3. Coat the ribs all over with mustard and season them with the rub. Using your two hands, work with the rub into the meat.

4. Put your ribs directly on the grill grate and smoke until their internal temperature reaches between 190°F and 200°F.

5. Remove the racks from the grill and cut them into individual ribs. Serve immediately.

Nutrition: Calories: 230 Carbs: 0g Fat: 17g Protein: 20g

51. Herbed Beef Eye Fillet

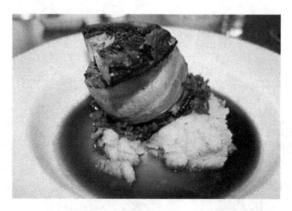

Preparation Time: 15 minutes

Cooking Time: 8 hours

Servings: 6

Ingredients:

- Pepper

- Salt

- Two tablespoons chopped rosemary

- Two tablespoons chopped basil

- Two tablespoons olive oil

- Three cloves crushed garlic

- ¼ cup chopped oregano

- ¼ cup chopped parsley

- 2 pounds beef eye fillet

Directions:

1. Use salt and pepper to rub in the meat before placing it in a container.

2. Place the garlic, oil, rosemary, oregano, basil, and parsley in a bowl. Stir well to combine.

3. Rub the fillet generously with this mixture on all sides. Let the meat sit on the counter for 30 minutes.

4. Add wood pellets to your smoker and follow your cooker's startup procedure. Preheat your smoker, with your lid closed, until it reaches 450.

5. Lay the meat on the grill, cover, and smoke for ten minutes per side or your preferred tenderness.

6. Once it is done to your likeness, allow it to rest for ten minutes. Slice and enjoy.

Nutrition: Calories: 202 Carbs: 0g Fat: 8g Protein: 33g

52. Beer Honey Steaks

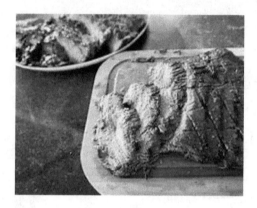

Preparation Time: 10 minutes

Cooking Time: 55 minutes

Servings: 4

Ingredients:

- Pepper

- Juice of one lemon

- 1 cup beer of choice

- One tablespoon honey

- Salt

- Two tablespoons olive oil

- One teaspoon thyme

- Four steaks of choice

Directions:

1. Season the steaks with pepper and salt.

2. Combine the olive oil, lemon juice, honey, thyme, and beer.

3. Rub the steaks with this mixture generously.

4. Add wood pellets to your smoker and follow your cooker's startup procedure. Preheat your smoker, with your lid closed, until it reaches 450.

5. Place the steaks onto the grill, cover, and smoke for ten minutes per side.

6. For about 10 minutes, let it cool after removing it from the grill.

Nutrition: Calories: 245 Carbs: 8gFat: 5g Protein: 40g

Fish Seafood Recipes

53. Sweet Honey Soy Smoked Salmon

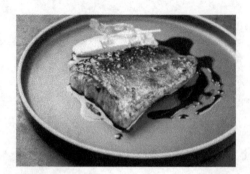

Preparation time: 15 minutes

Cooking time: 2 hours and 10 minutes

Servings: 10

Ingredients:

- Salmon fillet (4-lbs., 1.8-kg.)

The Brine:

- ¾ cup Brown sugar

- 3 tbsp. Soy sauce

- 3 tsp. Kosher salt

- 3 cups Coldwater

The Glaze:

- 2 tbsp. Butter

- 2 tbsp. Brown sugar

- 2 tbsp. Olive oil

- 2 tbsp. Honey

- 1 tbsp. Soy sauce

The Heat:

- Alder wood pellets

Directions:

1. Add brown sugar, soy sauce, and kosher salt to the cold water, then stir until dissolved.

2. Put the salmon fillet into the brine mixture and soak it for at least 2 hours.

3. After 2 hours, take the salmon fillet out of the brine, then wash and rinse it.

4. Plug the wood pellet smoker and place the wood pellet inside the hopper. Turn the switch on.

5. Set the temperature to 225°F (107°C) and prepare the wood pellet smoker for indirect heat. Wait until the wood pellet smoker is ready.

6. Place the salmon fillet in the wood pellet smoker and smoke it for 2 hours.

7. In the meantime, melt the butter over low heat, then mix it with brown sugar, olive oil, honey, and soy sauce. Mix well.

8. After an hour of smoking, baste the glaze mixture over the salmon fillet and repeat it once every 10 minutes.

9. Smoke until the salmon is flaky and remove it from the wood pellet smoker.

10. Transfer the smoked salmon fillet to a serving dish and baste the remaining glaze mixture over it.

11. Serve and enjoy.

Nutrition:

- Amount per 199 g

- = 1 serving(s)

- Energy (calories): 345 kcal

- Protein: 37.42 g

- Fat: 15.6 g

- Carbohydrates: 11.52 g

54. Cranberry Lemon Smoked Mackerel

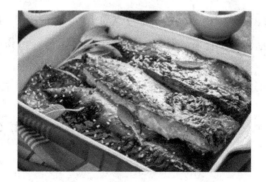

Preparation time: 15 minutes

Cooking time: 2 hours and 10 minutes

Servings: 10

Ingredients:

- Mackerel fillet (3.5-lb., 2.3-kg.)

The Brine:

- Three cans of cranberry juice

- ½ cup pineapple juice

- 3 cups cold water

- ¼ cup brown sugar

- Two cinnamon stick

- Two fresh lemons

- Two bay leaves

- Three fresh thyme leaves

The Rub:

- ¾ tsp. kosher salt

- ¾ tsp. pepper

The Heat:

- Alder wood pellets

Directions:

1. Mix the cranberry juice and pineapple juice with water, then stir well.

2. Stir in brown sugar to the liquid mixture, then mix until dissolved.

3. Cut the lemons into slices, then add them to the liquid mixture and cinnamon sticks, bay leaves, and fresh thyme leaves.

4. Put the mackerel fillet into the brine and soak it for at least 2 hours. Store it in the refrigerator to keep the mackerel fillet fresh.

5. After 2 hours, remove the mackerel fillet from the refrigerator and take it out of the brine mixture.

6. Plug the wood pellet smoker and place the wood pellet inside the hopper. Turn the switch on.

7. Set the temperature to 225°F (107°C) and prepare the wood pellet smoker for indirect heat. Wait until the wood pellet smoker is ready.

8. Sprinkle salt and pepper over the mackerel fillet, then place it in the wood pellet smoker.

9. Smoke the mackerel fillet for 2 hours or until it flakes and removes it from the wood pellet smoker.

10. Transfer the smoked mackerel fillet to a serving dish and serve.

11. Enjoy!

Nutrition:

- Amount per 225 g

- = 1 serving(s)

- Energy (calories): 386 kcal

- Protein: 46.11 g

- Fat: 4.56 g

- Carbohydrates: 37.85 g

55. Citrusy Smoked Tuna Belly with Sesame Aro

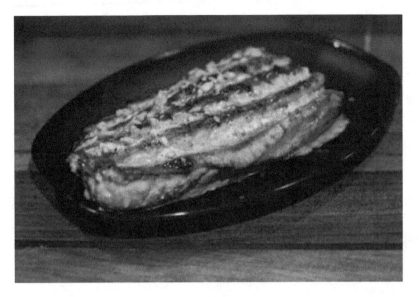

Preparation time: 15 minutes

Cooking time: 2 hours and 10 minutes

Servings: 10

Ingredients:

- Tuna belly (4-lbs., 1.8-kg.)

The Marinade:

- 3 tbsp. sesame oil

- ½ cup of soy sauce

- 2 tbsp. lemon juice

- ½ cup of orange juice

- 2 tbsp. Chopped fresh parsley

- ½ tsp. oregano

- 1 tbsp. minced garlic

- 2 tbsp. brown sugar

- 1 tsp. Kosher salt

- ½ tsp. pepper

The Glaze:

- 2 tbsp. maple syrup

- 1 tbsp. balsamic vinegar

The Heat:

- Mesquite wood pellets

Directions:

1. Combine sesame oil with soy sauce, lemon juice, and orange juice, then mix well.

2. Add oregano, minced garlic, brown sugar, kosher salt, pepper, chopped parsley to the wet mixture, and then stir until incorporated.

3. Carefully apply the wet mixture over the tuna fillet and marinate it for 2 hours. Store it in the refrigerator to keep the tuna fresh.

4. After 2 hours, remove the marinated tuna from the wood pellet smoker and thaw it at room temperature.

5. Plug the wood pellet smoker and place the wood pellet inside the hopper. Turn the switch on.

6. Set the temperature to 225°F (107°C) and prepare the wood pellet smoker for indirect heat. Wait until the wood pellet smoker is ready.

7. Place the marinated tuna fillet in the wood pellet smoker and smoke it until flaky.

8. Once it is done, remove the smoked tuna fillet from the wood pellet smoker and transfer it to a serving dish.

9. Mix the maple syrup with balsamic vinegar, then baste the mixture over the smoked tuna fillet.

10. Serve and enjoy.

Nutrition:

- Amount per 195 g

- = 1 serving(s)

- Energy (calories): 206 kcal

- Protein: 35.84 g

- Fat: 4.96 g

- Carbohydrates: 4.98 g

56. Savory Smoked Trout with Fennel and Black Pepper Rub

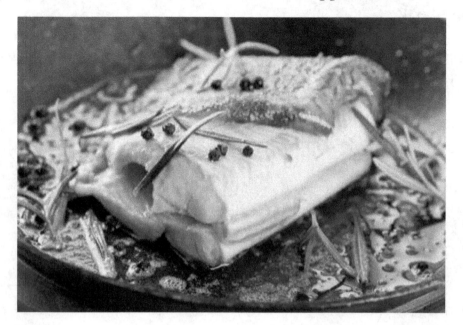

Preparation time: 15 minutes

Cooking time: 2 hours 10 minutes

Servings: 10

Ingredients:

- Trout fillet (4,5-lb., 2.3-kg.)

The Rub:

- 2 tbsp. lemon juice

- 3 tbsp. fennel seeds

- 1 ½ tbsp. ground coriander

- 1 tbsp. Black pepper

- ½ tsp. chili powder

- 1 tsp. kosher salt

- 1 tsp. garlic powder

The Glaze:

- 3 tbsp. olive oil

The Heat:

- Mesquite wood pellets

Directions:

1. Drizzle lemon juice over the trout fillet and let it rest for approximately 10 minutes.

2. In the meantime, combine the fennel seeds with coriander, black pepper, chili powder, salt, and garlic powder, then mix well.

3. Rub the trout fillet with the spice mixture, then set aside.

4. Plug the wood pellet smoker and place the wood pellet inside the hopper. Turn the switch on.

5. Set the temperature to 225°F (107°C) and prepare the wood pellet smoker for indirect heat. Wait until the wood pellet smoker is ready.

6. Place the seasoned trout fillet in the wood pellet smoker and smoke it for 2 hours.

7. Baste olive oil over the trout fillet and repeat it once every 20 minutes.

8. Once the smoked trout flakes, remove it from the wood pellet smoker and transfer it to a serving dish.

9. Serve and enjoy.

Nutrition:

- Energy (calories): 185 kcal

- Protein: 47.32 g

- Fat: 17.18 g

- Carbohydrates: 0.94 g

57. Sweet Smoked Shrimps Garlic Butter

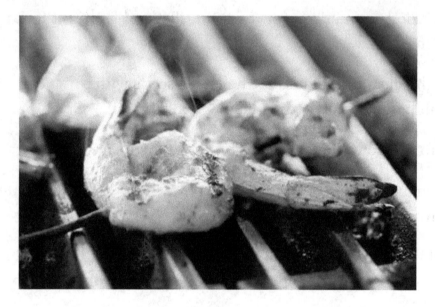

Preparation time: 15 minutes

Cooking time: 20 minutes

Servings: 10

Ingredients:

- Fresh shrimps (2-lbs., 0.9-kg.)

The Rub:

- 2 tbsp. Lemon juice

- ½ tsp. Salt

- ½ tsp. Black pepper

The Glaze:

- 2 tbsp. Butter

- ½ tsp. Garlic powder

The Heat:

- Hickory wood pellets

Directions:

1. Peel the fresh shrimps and drizzle lemon juice over them. Let them rest for several minutes.

2. After that, sprinkle salt and black pepper over the shrimps and spread them in a disposable aluminum pan.

3. Plug the wood pellet smoker and place the wood pellet inside the hopper. Turn the switch on.

4. Set the temperature to 200°F (93°C) and prepare the wood pellet smoker for indirect heat. Wait until the wood pellet smoker is ready.

5. Insert the aluminum pan with shrimps into the wood pellet smoker and smoke the shrimps for approximately 20 minutes.

6. Regularly check the shrimps and once they turn pink, take them out of the wood pellet smoker.

7. Add garlic powder to the butter, then mix until combined. The butter will be soft.

8. Baste the garlic butter over the smoked shrimps and serve.

9. Enjoy!

Nutrition:

- Amount per 94 g

- = 1 serving(s)

- Energy (calories): 99 kcal

- Protein: 18.6 g

- Fat: 2.01 g

- Carbohydrates: 0.21 g

58. Spiced Smoked Crabs with Lemon Grass

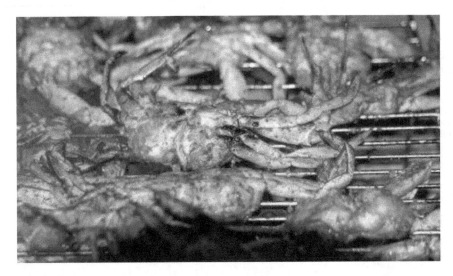

Preparation time: 15 minutes

Cooking time: 20 minutes

Servings: 10

Ingredients:

- Fresh crabs (5-lb., 2.3-kg.)

The Rub:

- 2 tbsp. smoked paprika

- 1 tsp. kosher salt

- 2 tbsp. dried parsley

- 2 tbsp. dried thyme

- 1 tbsp. black pepper

- 1 tsp. cayenne pepper

- 1 tsp. Allspice

- ½ tsp. Ground ginger

- ½ tsp. cinnamon powder

- Two lemongrass

The Heat:

- Hickory wood pellets

Directions:

1. Combine the smoked paprika, salt, parsley, thyme, black pepper, ground ginger, cinnamon powder, cayenne pepper, and allspice, then mix well.

2. Arrange the crabs in a disposable aluminum pan, then sprinkle the spice mixture over them.

3. Add lemongrasses on top, then cover the seasoned crabs with aluminum foil.

4. Plug the wood pellet smoker and place the wood pellet inside the hopper. Turn the switch on.

5. Set the temperature to 200°F (93°C) and prepare the wood pellet smoker for indirect heat. Wait until the wood pellet smoker is ready.

6. Insert the aluminum pan with crabs into the wood pellet smoker and smoke the crabs for 30 minutes.

7. Once it is done, take the smoked crabs out of the wood pellet smoker and serve.

8. Enjoy!

Nutrition:

- Amount per 229 g

- = 1 serving(s)

- Energy (calories): 201 kcal

- Protein: 41.14 g

- Fat: 2.58 g

- Carbohydrates: 0.98 g

59. Tequila Orange Marinade Smoked Lobster

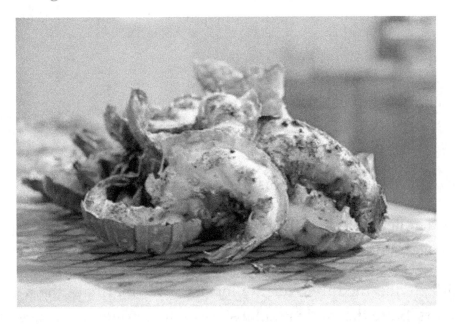

Preparation time: 15 minutes

Cooking time: 1 hour 10 minutes

Servings: 10

Ingredients:

- Fresh lobsters (5-lb., 2.3-kg.)

The Marinade:

- ¼ cup Tequila

- 3 tbsp. Lemon juice

- Two cups Orange juice

- ½ tsp. Grated lemon zest

- ½ tsp. Grated orange zest

- 1 tsp. Kosher salt

- ¼ tsp. Pepper

The Heat:

- Hickory wood pellets

Directions:

1. Mix the tequila with lemon juice and orange juice, then stir well.

2. Add grated lemon zest, orange zest, salt, and pepper to the liquid mixture, then stir until dissolved.

3. Drizzle the mixture over the lobsters and marinate them for at least 2 hours. Store the marinated lobsters in the refrigerator to keep them fresh.

4. After 2 hours, take the marinated lobsters out of the refrigerator and thaw them at room temperature.

5. Plug the wood pellet smoker and place the wood pellet inside the hopper. Turn the switch on.

6. Set the temperature to 200°F (93°C) and prepare the wood pellet smoker for indirect heat. Wait until the wood pellet smoker is ready.

7. Arrange the marinated lobsters in the wood pellet smoker and smoke them for an hour or until the smoked lobsters' internal temperature reaches 145°F (63°C).

8. Remove the smoked lobsters from the wood pellet smoker and transfer them to a serving dish.

9. Serve and enjoy.

Nutrition:

- Amount per 192 g

- = 1 serving(s)

- Energy (calories): 189 kcal

- Protein: 37.66 g

- Fat: 1.74 g

- Carbohydrates: 3.42 g

60. Beer Butter Smoked Clams

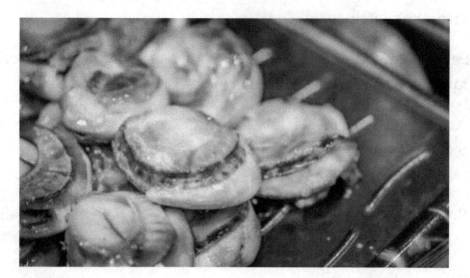

Preparation time: 15 minutes

Cooking time: 30 minutes

Servings: 10

Ingredients:

- Fresh clams (5-lb., 2.3-kg.)

The Sauce:

- One bottle beer

- 2 tbsp. olive oil

- 2 tbsp. minced garlic

- 1 tsp. salt

- ¼ cup butter

The Heat:

- Hickory wood pellets

Directions:

1. Preheat a saucepan over medium heat, then pour olive oil into it.

2. Once the oil is hot, stir in the minced garlic and sauté until wilted and aromatic.

3. Remove the saucepan from heat, then pour beer into it.

4. Add salt to the mixture, then stir until incorporated.

5. Spread the clams in a disposable aluminum pan, then pour the beer mixture over the clams.

6. Drop butter at several places on top of the clams, then set aside.

7. Plug the wood pellet smoker and place the wood pellet inside the hopper. Turn the switch on.

8. Set the temperature to 200°F (93°C) and prepare the wood pellet smoker for indirect heat. Wait until the wood pellet smoker is ready.

9. Insert the aluminum pan with clams into the wood pellet smoker and smoke the clams for half an hour.

10. Once it is done and the smoked clams' shells are open, take them out of the wood pellet smoker.

11. Transfer the smoked clams to a serving dish and enjoy.

Nutrition:

- Amount per 138 g

- = 1 serving(s)

- Energy (calories): 137 kcal

- Protein: 1.51 g

- Fat: 3.41 g

- Carbohydrates: 25.12 g

61. Bbq Oysters

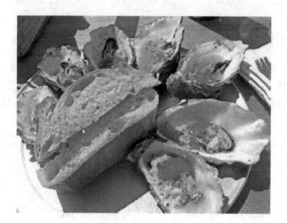

Servings: 4-6

Cooking Time: 16 Minutes

Ingredients:

- Shucked oysters - 12

- Unsalted butter - 1 lb.

- Chopped green onions - 1 bunch

- Honey Hog BBQ Rub or Meat Church "The Gospel" - 1 tbsp

- Minced green onions - ½ bunch

- Seasoned breadcrumbs - ½ cup

- Cloves of minced garlic - 2

- Shredded pepper jack cheese - 8 oz

- Heat and Sweet BBQ sauce

Directions:

1. Preheat the pellet grill for about 10-15 minutes with the lid closed.

2. To make the compound butter, wait for the butter to soften. Then combine the butter, onions, BBQ rub, and garlic thoroughly.

3. Lay the butter evenly on plastic wrap or parchment paper. Roll it up in a log shape and tie the ends with butcher's twine. Place these in the freezer to solidify for an hour. This butter can be used on any kind of grilled meat to enhance its flavor. Any other high-quality butter can also replace this compound butter.

4. Shuck the oysters, keeping the juice in the shell.

5. Sprinkle all the oysters with breadcrumbs and place them directly on the grill. Allow them to cook for 5 minutes. You will know they are cooked when the oysters begin to curl slightly at the edges.

6. Once they are cooked, put a spoonful of the compound butter on the oysters. Once the butter melts, you can add a little bit of pepper jack cheese to add more flavor to them.

7. The oysters must not be on the grill for longer than 6 minutes, or you risk overcooking them. Put a generous squirt of the BBQ sauce on all the oysters. Also, add a few chopped onions.

8. Allow them to cool for a few minutes and enjoy the taste of the sea!

Nutrition Info: Carbohydrates: 2.5 g Protein: 4.7 g Fat: 1.1 g Sodium: 53 mg Cholesterol: 25 mg

62. Blackened Catfish

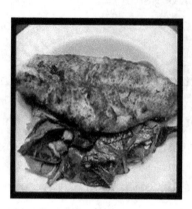

Servings: 4

Cooking Time: 40 Minutes

Ingredients:

- Spice blend

- 1teaspoon granulated garlic

- 1/4 teaspoon cayenne pepper

- 1/2 cup Cajun seasoning

- 1teaspoon ground thyme

- 1teaspoon ground oregano

- 1teaspoon onion powder

- 1tablespoon smoked paprika

- 1teaspoon pepper

- Fish

- 4 catfish fillets

- Salt to taste

- 1/2 cup butter

Directions:

1. In a bowl, combine all the ingredients for the spice blend.

2. Sprinkle both sides of the fish with the salt and spice blend.

3. Set your wood pellet grill to 450 degrees F.

4. Heat your cast iron pan and add the butter. Add the fillets to the pan.

5. Cook for 5 minutes per side.

6. Serving Suggestion: Garnish with lemon wedges.

7. Tip: Smoke the catfish for 20 minutes before seasoning.

Nutrition Info: Calories: 181.5 Fat: 10.5 g Cholesterol: 65.8 mg Carbohydrates: 2.9 g Fiber: 1.8 g Sugars: 0.4 g Protein: 19.2 g

63. Grilled Shrimp

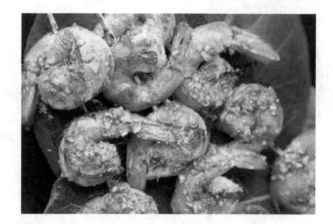

Servings: 4

Cooking Time: 15 Minutes

Ingredients:

- Jumbo shrimp peeled and cleaned - 1 lb.

- Oil - 2 tbsp

- Salt - ½ tbsp

- Skewers - 4-5

- Pepper - ⅛ tbsp

- Garlic salt - ½ tbsp

Directions:

1. Preheat the wood pellet grill to 375 degrees.

2. Mix all the ingredients in a small bowl.

3. After washing and drying the shrimp, mix it well with the oil and seasonings.

4.   Add skewers to the shrimp and set the bowl of shrimp aside.

5.   Open the skewers and flip them.

6.   Cook for four more minutes. Remove when the shrimp is opaque and pink.

Nutrition Info: Carbohydrates: 1.3 g Protein: 19 g Fat: 1.4 g Sodium: 805 mg Cholesterol: 179 mg

64. Grilled Lobster Tail

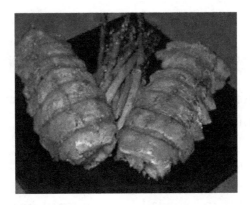

Servings: 4

Cooking Time: 15 Minutes

Ingredients:

- 2 (8 ounces each) lobster tails

- 1/4 tsp old bay seasoning

- ½ tsp oregano

- 1 tsp paprika

- Juice from one lemon

- 1/4 tsp Himalayan salt

- 1/4 tsp freshly ground black pepper

- 1/4 tsp onion powder

- 2 tbsp freshly chopped parsley

- ¼ cup melted butter

Directions:

1. Slice the tail in the middle with a kitchen shear. Pull the shell apart slightly and run your hand through the meat to separate the meat partially

2. Combine the seasonings

3. Drizzle lobster tail with lemon juice and season generously with the seasoning mixture.

4. Preheat your wood pellet smoker to 450°F using applewood pellets.

5. Place the lobster tail directly on the grill grate, meat side down. Cook for about 15 minutes.

6. The tails must be pulled off, and it must cool down for a few minutes

7. Drizzle melted butter over the tails.

8. Serve and garnish with fresh chopped parsley.

Nutrition Info: Calories: 146 Cal Fat: 11.7 g Carbohydrates: 2.1 g Protein: 9.3 g Fiber: 0.8 g

65. Stuffed Shrimp Tilapia

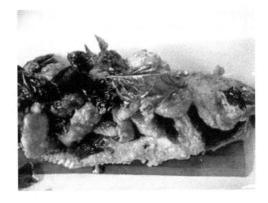

Servings: 5

Cooking Time: 45 Minutes

Ingredients:

- 5 ounces fresh, farmed tilapia fillets

- 2 tablespoons extra virgin olive oil

- 1and ½ teaspoons smoked paprika

- 1and ½ teaspoons Old Bay seasoning

- Shrimp stuffing

- 1pound shrimp, cooked and deveined

- 1tablespoon salted butter

- 1cup red onion, diced

- 1cup Italian bread crumbs

- ½ cup mayonnaise

- 1large egg, beaten

- 2teaspoons fresh parsley, chopped

- 1and ½ teaspoons salt and pepper

Directions:

1. Take a food processor and add shrimp, chop them up

2. Take a skillet and place it over medium-high heat, add butter and allow it to melt

3. Sauté the onions for 3 minutes

4. Add chopped shrimp with cooled Sautéed onion alongside remaining ingredients listed under stuffing ingredients and transfer to a bowl

5. Cover the mixture and allow it to refrigerate for 60 minutes

6. Rub both sides of the fillet with olive oil

7. Spoon 1/3 cup of the stuffing into the fillet

8. Flatten out the stuffing onto the bottom half of the fillet and fold the Tilapia in half

9. Secure with two toothpicks

10. Dust each fillet with smoked paprika and Old Bay seasoning

11. Preheat your smoker to 400 degrees Fahrenheit

12. Add your preferred wood Pellets and transfer the fillets to a non-stick grill tray

13. Transfer to your smoker and smoker for 30-45 minutes until the internal temperature reaches 145 degrees Fahrenheit

14. Allow the fish to rest for 5 minutes and enjoy!

Nutrition Info: Calories: 620 Fats: 50g Carbs: 6g Fiber: 1g

66. Grilled Shrimp Kabobs

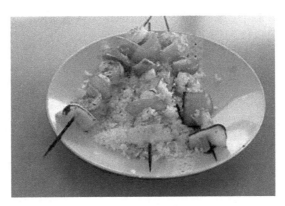

Servings: 4

Cooking Time: 10 Minutes

Ingredients:

- 1 lb. colossal shrimp, peeled and deveined

- 2 tbsp. oil

- 1/2 tbsp. garlic salt

- 1/2 tbsp. salt

- 1/8 tbsp. pepper

- 6 skewers

Directions:

1. Preheat your to 375F.

2. Pat the shrimp dry with a paper towel.

3. In a mixing bowl, mix oil, garlic salt, salt, and pepper

4. Toss the shrimp in the mixture until well coated.

5. Skewer the shrimps and cook in with the lid closed for 4 minutes.

6. Open the lid, flip the skewers, cook for another 4 minutes, or wait until the shrimp is pink and the flesh is opaque.

7. Serve.

Nutrition Info: Calories 325, Total fat 0g, Saturated fat 0g, Total carbs 5g, Net carbs 2g Protein 20g, Sodium 120mg

67. Wood Pellet Grilled Lobster Tail

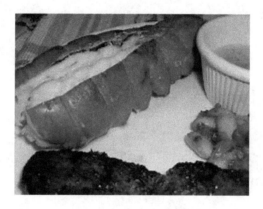

Servings: 2

Cooking Time: 15 Minutes

Ingredients:

- 10 oz lobster tail

- 1/4 tbsp old bay seasoning

- 1/4 tbsp Himalayan sea salt

- 2 tbsp butter, melted

- 1 tbsp fresh parsley, chopped

Directions:

1. Preheat the wood pellet to 450°F.

2. Slice the tails down the middle using a knife.

3. Season with seasoning and salt, then place the tails on the grill grate.

4. Grill for 15 minutes or until the internal temperature reaches 140°F.

5. Remove the tails and drizzle with butter and garnish with parsley.

6. Serve and enjoy.

Nutrition Info: Calories 305, Total fat 14g, Saturated fat 12g, Total Carbs 10g, Net Carbs 5g, Protein 20g, Sodium: 690mg, Potassium 165mg

68. Buttered Crab Legs

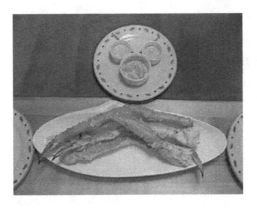

Servings: 4

Cooking Time: 10 Minutes

Ingredients:

- 12 tablespoons butter

- One tablespoon parsley, chopped

- One tablespoon tarragon, chopped

- One tablespoon chives, chopped

- One tablespoon lemon juice

- 4 lb. king crab legs, split in the center

Directions:

1. Set the wood pellet grill to 375 degrees F.

2. Preheat it for 15 minutes while the lid is closed.

3. In a pan over medium heat, simmer the butter, herbs, and lemon juice for 2 minutes.

4. Place the crab legs on the grill.

5. Pour half of the sauce on top.

6. Grill for 10 minutes.

7. Serve with the reserved butter sauce.

8. Tips: You can also use shrimp for this recipe.

69. Citrus Salmon

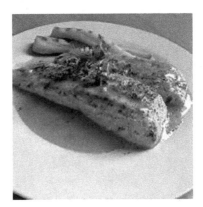

Servings: 6

Cooking Time: 30 Minutes

Ingredients:

- 2 (1-lb.) salmon fillets

- Salt and freshly ground black pepper, to taste

- 1 tbsp. seafood seasoning

- 2 lemons, sliced

- 2 limes, sliced

Directions:

1. Set the Grill temperature to 225 degrees F and preheat with a closed lid for 15 minutes.

2. Season the salmon fillets with salt, black pepper, and seafood seasoning evenly.

3. Place the salmon fillets onto the grill and top each with lemon and lime slices evenly.

4.   Cook for about 30 minutes.

5.   Remove the salmon fillets from the grill and serve hot.

Nutrition Info: Calories per serving: 327; Carbohydrates: 1g; Protein: 36.1g; Fat: 19.8g; Sugar: 0.2g; Sodium: 237mg; Fiber: 0.3g

70. Barbecued Scallops

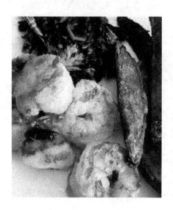

Servings: 4

Cooking Time: 10 Minutes

Ingredients:

- 1 pound large scallops

- 2 tablespoons olive oil

- 1 batch Dill Seafood Rub

Directions:

1.   Supply your smoker with wood pellets and follow the manufacturer's specific start-up procedure. Preheat the grill, with the lid closed, to 375°F.

2. Coat the scallops all over with olive oil and season all sides with the rub.

3. Place the scallops directly on the grill grate and grill for 5 minutes per side. Remove the scallops from the grill and serve immediately.

Conclusion

The Pit Boss Wood Pellet Grill is a popular grill of 2019 that features a large cooking area, dual venting for temperature control, and an easy-to-use digital controller.

It is a great tool for smoking your favorite foods. Well, it is fortunate that this grill can smoke your meat evenly and effectively.

The manufacturer uses only superior quality materials to make it possible for you to cook different kinds of food. It has a large cooking area, which means you can use it for different parties or gatherings. It is a great tool for entertaining your friends and families.

We hope that this guide will help you in your quest for the perfect summertime cookout. Thanks to our tips and tricks, you'll be able to take your grilling and smoking skills from mediocre to masterful with just a little patience.

No more greasy fingers! No more dishpan hands! And no more burnt barbecue nightmares. Throw a party any time with these stick-handled recipes, the best barbecue sauces we've ever tried, and our secret weapon: The PIT BOSS WOOD PELLET GRILL & SMOKER COOKBOOK.

We encourage you to share these tips and recipes with your friends and neighbors. Due to the rising popularity of wood pellet grills, we hope that many will switch from propane to hardwood. When they do, help them get started in the right direction by sharing this recipe book.

The Carnivore Meal Plan Cookbook for Athletes

The Protein-Based Program You Need to Build Progressive Endurance and Strength like a Pro [Meal Plan Worth: 1.375$]

By

Chef Marcello Ruby

Contents

INTRODUCTION **146**

CHAPTER 1: WHAT IS THE CARNIVORE DIET? **148**

1.1 HOW TO ORGANIZE YOUR MEAL PLAN FOR YOUR CARNIVORE DIET 149

1.2 15 DAYS MEAL PLAN FOR THE CARNIVORE DIET 152

1.3 WHAT FOOD IS INCLUDED IN THE CARNIVORE DIET? 157

1.4 WHAT FOOD ITEMS AVOIDED ON THE CARNIVORE DIET? 158

1.5 HOW CARNIVORE DIETS HAVE BENEFICIAL EFFECTS? 160

1.6 SIDE EFFECTS OF CARNIVORE DIET AND THEIR CURES? 166

CHAPTER 2: BREAKFAST RECIPES FOR THE CARNIVORE DIET **173**

1. CARNIVORE BREAKFAST SANDWICH 173

2. CHEESY 3-MEAT BREAKFAST CASSEROLE RECIPE 175

3. ONE-PAN EGG AND TURKEY SKILLET RECIPE 177

4. KETO AND CARNIVORE MEATLOAF MUFFIN 178

5. CARNIVORE KETO BURGERS 180

6 LOW-CARB BAKED EGGS 182

7. SPAM AND EGGS 184

CHAPTER 3: LUNCH RECIPES FOR CARNIVORE DIET **186**

1. CARNIVORE CHICKEN NUGGETS 186

2. CHEESY AIR FRYER MEATBALLS 188

3. SCALLOPS WITH WRAPPED BACON 190

4. STEAK TARTARE 191

5. LOW-CARB BEEF BOURGUIGNON STEW 193

6. LUNCH MEAT ROLL-UPS 198

7. CARNIVORE BRAISED BEEF SHANK 199

8. HERB ROASTED BONE MARROW 202

CHAPTER 4: DESSERTS AND SNACK RECIPES FOR THE CARNIVORE DIET

....204

1. BACONY CARNIVORE WOMELLETES 204

2. CARNIVORE CAKE 205

3. EGG CUSTARD 207

4. CARNIVORE CHAFFLE RECIPE 209

5. MEAT BAGELS 212

CHAPTER 5: DINNER RECIPES FOR THE CARNIVORE DIET 214

1. POT ROAST RECIPE WITH GRAVY 214

2. CARNIVORE SKILLET PEPPERONI PIZZA 217

3. CARNIVORE HAM AND CHEESE NOODLE SOUP 219

4. CARNIVORE MOUSSAKA 220

5. AIP CHICKEN BACON SAUTÉ 223

6. LOW CARB CARNITAS 225

7. CARNIVORE'S LASAGNA 227

CONCLUSION 231

Introduction

Nutrition is crucial for athletes at the most fundamental level because it offers an energy source to conduct the task. Our power, preparation, productivity, and training are influenced by the meal we intake. Not only is the kind of food important to sports nutrition, but the times we consume across the day also affect our levels of performance and the ability of our bodies to recover after exercise. It's important to set your goals before you start eating the carnivorous diet method.

Keep in mind this is a change in lifestyle - no carbs, no plants, only products from animals and lots of good fat. You need to know why you are getting into the carnivore diet throughout the first place, whether it's to achieve your intended body weight, fight food allergies, decrease body fat battle with an autoimmune condition, and construct some muscular strength.

The Carnivore Diet arises from the widespread concept that mainly meat and fish were consumed by human ancestor communities and that high-carb diets are responsible for today's high rates of infectious disease.

Meals ingested before and after the workout are the most important thing about sports performance, but you should always be vigilant with all you put into your body. Athletes should eat around two hours before practicing as a general rule, and this diet should be low in fat, high in carbohydrates and high in protein.

The primary source of nutrition that drives your exercise schedule is protein, and carbohydrates are needed to help muscle recovery. You, therefore, need to replace the nutrients you have lost after exercising, and by incorporating protein in your post-workout meal, you need to allow consistent muscle recovery.

Chapter 1: What is the carnivore diet?

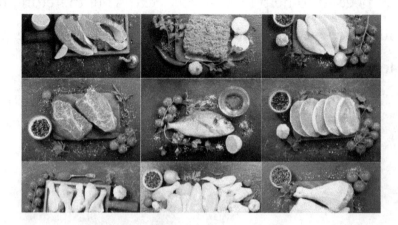

The Carnivore diet consists of foods dependent on animals, including fish, meat, low lactose milk and eggs products. Honey, zero carb seasoning, salt and pepper may also be used by a consumer pursuing the diet.

Certain items are eliminated from the diet, like grains, vegetables and fruits, plant-based oils, high lactose milk and carbohydrates.

The carnivore diet is based on the controversial theory that it was rich in meat eaten by human ancestors long ago. It assumes that when boosted by high protein and fat levels, human bodies operate best.

Figures such as Jordan Peterson (bestselling author and psychologist), Joe Rogan (standup comedian and podcast host), Shawn Baker (retired orthopedic surgeon) have made the diet popular.

On Carnivore Diet, once the appetite is satisfied, you eat fatty cuts of the high-quality meal and avoid all carbs, Sauces, Fruits, Nuts, Plant-based food, and Veggies.

Therefore, a carnivore diet is considered an "elimination diet" that can clarify its effectiveness in supporting others with digestive issues, constipation, and food sensitivities.

71. 1.1 How to organize your meal plan for your Carnivore Diet.

In Carnivore Diet, these tips have enabled us a great deal to remain encouraged and accomplish some auxiliary goals. That's the opportunity to get rid of extra fat, lose weight and attain that little muscular strength without missing the micronutrients needed. So, get into it now.

1. Know Your Why

It's necessary to set your objectives before you start your carnivore diet plan. Note that it is indeed a shift of lifestyle no carbs, no plants, just products from animals and lots of healthy fat. You have to remember why you are going into a carnivore diet from the first place, whether it's to achieve your target body weight, decrease body fat, battle digestive problems, cure an autoimmune condition, or create some lean muscle.

Depending on your needs, you have to assign yourself a clear goal. Perhaps it's about losing 20 lbs. Whether you go out on a summer break and acquire 5 pounds of muscle mass in six months - whatever it is, in the entire process, Stay close to the meat-only diet style.

It would be like a suggestion to help you stay on track to proceed with the carnivore diet. Whatever that is, to inform you of your diet pattern, experienced carnivore dieters may write it all down and upload it somewhere that you can see each day. Based on your losing weight and other fitness objectives, it'll be like a way to remind you to keep you active to proceed with the carnivore diet.

2. Plan for sticking to The Meal Plan

It requires absolute devotion and determination to consume a moderate animal fat, carnivore diet for further than a few days or weeks. On the carnivore diet, the worst thing you can do is start taking it day by day and postpone it until the morning to find out what you're going to eat next. Instead, set specific targets for the week, use a diet planner, and list carnivore diet foods to schedule what animal products to consume in advance.

We also involve items like how many runs and visits to the workout we do, as well as what we'll have with each meal for our regular carnivore diet, in addition to having a carnivore diet food chart.

You may take some further time to discover new kinds of varieties of meat products you may like and methods of preparation to introduce a little more variety to your menu of animal meat. To try more diet choices and taste new tastes, you can also try on eating fresh animal organs (such as heart or cow liver). You can benefit from meal delivery if you are not dependent on cooking your foods while on the diet weight loss diet. It's an efficient method to reignite your Carnivore diet, and most significantly, according to your body's needs, you receive quality meats, pork, or chicken meat.

3.Preparations toward social life

The reality is that, on a carnivore diet, eating at social events seems to be one of the most disturbing situations. If you eat at a dinner party like that and tell people how every day eats lunch at McDonald's, eat Donuts and dinner pizza, you're not going to be judged more by people.

Suppose you tell another person on the table that you are on a carnivore diet meal schedule, though, because it includes eating only animal fat, zero plant foods and red meat because of your favorite diet. In that case, the entire table is now shocking. There's a vegetarian at the table, and Heaven forbid, you won't hear another word of it. Firstly, tell people you are doing so because of multiple problems with food allergies, and determining the underlying reasons, you are sticking with a carnivore diet.

Generally, at the start, we don't like speaking regarding weight loss. You'll only get remarks from several people so with this way, such as: "You're totally crazy not to eat fruit and veg, and it's so stupid." The vegetarian at the table will also have a lot of fruitier nutritional vocabulary and a long discussion about the need to eat fruit and veggies to get more nutrition. In this scenario, we find that asking if they are associated with their fitness or yours is the only solution that helps? It fits us nine times in a row, and if you get yourself sitting beside the vegetarian, then change the topic to another one.

4. Dining Out

The pleasant deal for people upon this carnivore diet is with quality nutrition meats that will suit your needs; there are many places you can eat out. Eating at BBQ and steak restaurants is probably the best decision you can make. But make sure to avoid animal meats that are frozen. In the carnivorous weight loss diet, consuming meat products is not tolerated. Everything you need to do is pay attention to the way the meals are prepared. While on a carnivore diet, the main thing is to avoid consuming something that includes stir-fried vegetables or sauces.

Unfortunately, in many Indian and Chinese restaurants, you'll most likely stop eating out for a carnivore diet because almost all their meals are heavy with sauces and salt. What we usually do when we start our all-meat diet is review the menus online. We'd be likely to eat there as long as we see filet mignon and are steaks accessible.

1.2 15 days meal plan for the Carnivore Diet.

Carnivore Diet For 1st week

On Monday

Breakfast 1 or 2 100 percent pure pork sausages (3 ounces) and Five bacon slices (about 4 ounces)

Lunch just 10 ounces of grilled beef patty burger with a slice of cheese.

Dinner four stacks of healthy lamb (12 ounces)

On Tuesday

Breakfast 3 bacon slices (4 ounces) 3 grilled 100 percent pure pork sausages (about 5 ounces)

Lunch Slammed buttery cutlets of salmon upon the bone (about 15 ounces).

Dinner Porterhouse steak (12 ounces) grilled with butter.

On Wednesday

Breakfast Grilled trout fillets with butter (about 10 ounces)

Lunch Grilled belly of pork (about 10 ounces)

Dinner Slow beef roast upper side (about 12 ounces)

On Thursday

Breakfast Roasted ground beef burger patty with cheese (about 8 ounces)

Lunch Roast salmon cutlets with butter on the bone (about 15 ounces)

Dinner Grilled steak porterhouse (about 12 ounces)

On Friday

Breakfast 2 breasts of grilled chicken with skin (about 8 ounces)

Lunch fillets of fried trout (about 16 ounces)

Dinner Slow grilled upper side of beef (about 12 ounces)

On Saturday

Breakfast three 100 percent pure pork sausages grilled (about 5 ounces)

Lunch Three slices of bacon (about 4 ounces) Four healthy lamb chops (about 12 ounces)

Dinner Grilled steak ribeye (about 12 ounces)

On Sunday

Breakfast two breasts of grilled chicken with skin (about 8 ounces)

Lunch 4 grilled or fried pork chops (about 12 ounces)

Dinner Grilled steak ribeye (about 12 ounces)

Shopping list for 1st week

- Pork belly about 10 ounces

- Lamb Chops about 24 ounces

- Beef Grounded about eighteen ounces

- Porterhouse steak about twenty-four ounces

- Topside of beef about twenty-four ounces

- Salmon cutlets about thirty ounces (or other fatty fish)

- Trout about twenty-six ounces

- Butter around one lb.

- Cheese around half lbs.

- Bacon about twelve ounces

- 100 percent pork sausages around 13 ounces

- Pork chops about twelve ounces

- Chicken breasts

- Ribeye steak about twenty-four ounces

- The top side of beef about twenty-four ounces

- salmon cutlets about thirty ounces (or any other fish with fats)

Carnivore diet meal plan for 2nd week

We will be reducing much of the milk from items on our carnivore diet during the next week. We're still going to allow the butter to be utilized for the food, but dairy foods such as cheese will now be gone.

On Monday

Breakfast Two breasts of grilled chicken with skin (about 8 ounces)

Lunch Slow beef grilled topside (about 12 ounces)

Dinner four healthy lamb pieces (about 12 ounces)

Tuesday

Breakfast roasted ground beef patty burger (about 8 ounces)

Lunch on the bone roasted salmon cutlets (about 15 ounces)

Dinner Grilled steak ribeye (about 8 ounces) and roasted liver of beef (about 4 ounces)

On Wednesday

Breakfast 5 bacon slices (about 4 ounces) and one- or two-100 percent pork sausages (about 3 ounces)

Lunch grilled porterhouse steak with butter (about 12 ounces)

Dinner Slow beef roast topside (about 12 ounces)

On Thursday

Breakfast Grilled steak with ribeye (about 12 ounces)

Lunch 3 chicken breasts grilled with skin (around 12 ounces)

Dinner barbequed ground beef patty burger (around 12 ounces)

On Friday

Breakfast sirloin steak grilled with butter (about 8 ounces)

Lunch Slow beef roast topside (about 8 ounces) and roasted liver of beef (4 ounces)

Dinner with four fried or grilled pork pieces (about 12 ounces)

On Saturday

Breakfast Grilled ground beef patty burger (about 8 ounces)

Lunch Roast salmon cutlets on the bone with butter (about 15 ounces)

Dinner Grilled steak of sirloin (12 ounces)

On Sunday

Breakfast Grilled steak ribeye (about 8 ounces)

Lunch Slow roast beef upside (about 12 ounces)

Dinner 3 grilled with skin chicken breast (about 12 ounces) and roasted liver of beef (about 4 ounces)

Shopping list for 2nd week:

- Salmon cutlets about thirty ounces or any other fatty fish

- Ribeye steak about twenty-eight ounces

- Pork chops around twelve ounces

- Beef's liver around twelve ounces

- Ribeye steak around twenty-four ounces

- 100 percent pork sausages about three ounces

- Porterhouse steak about twelve ounces

- Chicken breasts about thirty-two ounces

- Topside of beef around forty-four ounces

- Lamb chops around twelve ounces

72. 1.3 What food is included in the carnivore diet?

The Carnivore Diet falls completely under one category of food: animal products.

Though animal products can break into additional categories, there are various content standards within each category. Now let's look into those classifications.

MEAT

Any type: lamb, beef, poultry, pork etc. Preferably choose grass-fed or organic meats.

ORGANS

Organs are an excellent substitute but are a key element of a well-formulated carnivore diet. Try to include chicken liver, kidneys, beef heart, beef liver, and brains.

EGGS.

Eggs of all kinds from most birds. Where possible, choose organic.

FISH AND SEAFOOD

Choose fatty fish such as sardines, mackerel, salmon herring are great and might even have health privilege due to high amounts of omega-3 fatty acids. Other seafood includes shrimp, squid tilapia, tuna, swordfish, and trout scallops.

DAIRY

Choose full-fat options where possible, like full-fat cream, real butter, sour cream, high-fat cheeses, and Greek yogurt. Try to use skim milk minimum, reduced fat, and regular milk as they contain many sugars.

FATS AND OILS

For cooking, use ghee, butter, tallow, lard, chicken fat, suet and tallow duck fat.

CARNIVORE DRINKS

WATER

Wherever appropriate, water must be your first preference. Try sparkling water if you think you're going to struggle with your water intake.

BONE BROTH

Broth from any animal's bones will make a drink that is warm and comforting.

TEA

Tea would Be OK with a drop of cream or milk. Green tea is best with no milk.

COFFEE

Coffee with milk, Black coffee or coffee with cream is all fine. Remember that the cream provides extra calories that you do not account for when attempting to lose weight.

73. 1.4 What Food items avoided on the Carnivore diet?

The Carnivore Diet prohibits all food that does not come from animals.

Restricted foods include:

Vegetables: green beans, cauliflower, potatoes, broccoli, peppers, etc.

Legumes: lentils, beans, etc.

Nuts and seeds: sunflower seeds, pumpkin seeds, almonds, pistachios, etc.

Grains: quinoa, bread, pasta, rice, wheat, etc.

Alcohol: wine, liquor, beer, etc.

Sugars: maple syrup, brown sugar, table sugar etc.

"Beverages" other than water: coffee, tea, fruit juice, soda etc.

PROCESSED MEATS

Process meats are highly insufficient in diet and moderate in chemical substances.

LOW-FAT MILK.

High sugar usually consists of skimmed milk and low fat. Unless you need to, restrict it to a few drops in your coffee or tea.

Sauces & Seasoning

While seasoning a steak with thyme, salt, or even paprika is not unusual, going too deep on sauces and seasoning can cause stomach issues for those with a weak immune system.

Foods on the Carnivore Diet that might be OK.

Foods that may be permissible include:

Milk

Yogurt

Cheese

74. 1.5 How carnivore diets have beneficial effects?

The carnivore diet has helped thousands of people fix the effects of many health conditions or improve them. Check out some favorable circumstances of the carnivore diet.

Minimize Acid Reflux

As stomach acid rises into the esophagus, acid reflux occurs, causing discomfort that can lead to heartburn symptoms. In the United States, this is relatively a common medical complaint, and many of us live on the belief that there is little we can do to change it. Fortunately, that isn't valid.

Although no food form has yet been shown to cure this disorder entirely, your dietary choices will help minimize or even eradicate symptoms a great deal. That makes a decent amount of sense, provided that in your stomach, this condition begins.

IMPROVED ACNE

Acne, defined by the occurrence of spots mostly on the face, neck and shoulders and is also a sign of hormonal changes that causes inflammation elsewhere in the body. It can be physically and psychologically uncomfortable, depending on your diet, and it's avoidable.

There are several reasons why the carnivore diet helps hold spots at bay. The key theory connects carbohydrate intake and acne. Image Inflammation is a significant cause of acne as well. Incidentally, in those that eat so many carbohydrates, inflammation is identified.

Meat also provides vital nutrients, which have also been observed to affect breakouts, including omega 3s and zinc. Several meat substitutes, such as milk, can also worsen no-ending acne. If you want flawless skin, a carnivore diet could provide an alternative.

Maintain ADD/ADHD

Hyperactivity disorders that affect kids, teenagers, and even adults are called ADD and ADHD. Either syndrome may contribute to hyperactivity, impaired control of impulses, and trouble paying attention.

It is no secret that in problems such as these, diet plays a major role. Although many studies of ADHD and diet effects are still needed, the wrong foods appear to worsen troublesome symptoms.

The advantages of the carnivore diet have been shown to improve the symptoms. Perhaps because of the interaction of plant foods with the gut microbiome.

PREVENT ALZHEIMER'S

Alzheimer's is a steady brain disease that kills memory, cognitive capacity, and comprehension of even basic activities such as brushing teeth. It has a devastating effect on the lives of patients affected and on their loved ones and sometimes results in hospitalization or treatment for the long term.

The good news is that there is evidence to indicate a diet that can help with such a carnivore diet free of plant foods. Although there is no way to reverse the effect of Alzheimer's, modifying diets like this might minimize symptoms. Studies show that consuming a lower diet of plant foods over your life can also minimize the risk of Alzheimer's by up to 44%!

The association between the lectins present in plants and Alzheimer's is the key explanation why plant foods are causing concern. As such, patients who eat large quantities of plant food can intensify their symptoms and put themselves at risk. By contrast, healthy fats such as those present in beef can hold symptoms at bay and, as a result, delay Alzheimer's expansion.

IMPROVE BLOOD PRESSURE

Blood pressure associate with the pressure of circulating blood on the walls of blood vessels. Lifestyle and diet control of blood pressure is essential for ongoing health and the prevention of progressive health problems such as heart disease. While meat gave a bad perspective when it comes to blood pressure, it is not reasonable.

In terms of blood pressure regulation, limiting carbohydrate intake and consuming red meat and fish, turkey, or skinless chicken have shown positive results.

It is mainly due to high levels of protein present in animal foods, according to studies. There is also some evidence that a balanced intake of vitamin D and omega-3 will help maintain an even keel for blood pressure rates. Obviously, with a very well carnivore diet, they are simple enough to come by.

REDUCE CANCER RISK

A disease that no one wishes to obtain is cancer, marked by the uncontrolled division of cancerous cells. It's one of the most serious diseases we struggle with without a cure today, despite medical advances and increased recovery rates.

Our chances of developing cancer will affect our lifestyle. Smoking, for instance, increases the probability of irregular cells. What fewer people know is that cancer and what we eat also have close ties. Although research is underway on exactly what effect food can have, a balanced diet is important to keep this problem at bay.

In particular, studies have shown that diets that are low in carbohydrates and rich in healthy proteins may help keep the body fit and resistant to cancer growth. Red meat and poultry can provide any diet with a great deal of protein while also maintaining gut bacteria as safe for cancer-fighting potential as possible.

DIABETES CONTROL

Diabetes is a chronic disorder that impacts the body's ability to maintain the consumption of sugar.

Type 1 diabetes happens when the body's immune system kills cells that contain insulin.

Type 2 diabetes happens when a person does not, in the first place, generate enough insulin. This disease, as you are probably aware, occurs mainly in people with low, high-sugar diets. In reality, by simply changing what they eat, some individuals with type 2 diabetes might completely turn around. Management of diabetes is a considerable health improvement of carnivore diet, and it is not unbelievable to see that high-quality meat may help minimize sugar intake. That's because the protein found in red meats will hold the level of satiety stable for longer, often without causing blood pressure to increase. Zero carbs, which has been proven to be one of the effective methods of controlling blood glucose levels, is also a carnivore diet.

WEIGHT LOSS

While we're on the topic of losing weight, the carnivore diet has become just another possible health gain. In the U.S. alone, estimates that there are approximately 160 million people above.

It is a set of problems because overweight itself can contribute to many of the issues we have addressed here, including heart diseases, thyroid issues, and diabetes. Fortunately, meat has one of the planet's most weight-loss-friendly ingredients. That's why the carnivore diet is so satisfying for so many.

Thanks to its high nutritional value, lean beef has specifically been found to be useful here. A high-quality steak will keep you energized, manage blood sugar, and also ensure that you don't need to have a snack. Protein was quite good for this; in particular, research has shown that a 25 percent increase in protein can reduce cravings by 60 percent. Even better, to appreciate those all-important advantages, you don't need to compromise on taste.

CONSTIPATION RELIEF

Constipation refers to irregular bodily functions that are hard to get through. What we eat will play a major role in producing symptoms in a condition of this type. And you can guarantee that when you spend all night in the bathroom, you will regret those unhealthy choices.

In contrast, it will help to keep our digestive system normal and flowing by shifting our preference to constipation-friendly menus. That, in turn, if we put the effort in, will hold the C-word at bay for our entire lives for a long period.

Here, the carnivore diet is also helpful as it offers delicious, low fiber meals that ensure that things move for you. No studies support the argument that high in fiber foods are beneficial for digestive health, and zero fiber diets have shown the best improvements in some research.

EPILEPSY MANAGEMENT

Epilepsy disrupts the mechanisms of brain messaging and thus causes frequent seizures. Some patients will only have seizures in their childhood and teenage years, whereas others will continue to fight epilepsy through their lifetime. Epilepsy causes fluctuate and may include head injuries and disorders of the brain. However, you might be surprised to learn that specialists have found proven advantages for patients concentrating on dietary changes, particularly low-carb diets such as the carnivore diet. Eating just meat may have such an effect that certain patients can decrease or eliminate drugs and encounter fewer or no seizures. In situations like this, high-fat products such as hamburgers and bacon also seem to have the best outcomes. Although it is not generally understood why all these foods have such a major effect on seizures (up to a reduction of 90%!), the research suggests that it can make a huge difference to eat more fat and to steer clear of carbohydrates.

Reduce THYROIDs Problems

Thyroid issues come in a variety of forms and often occur due to thyroid hormone production issues. The overproduction of certain hormones is hyperthyroidism. When the thyroid stops producing enough hormones, hypothyroidism occurs. Problems such as these can be dangerous for patients, although they are fully treatable with hormone substitutes or, in several cases, diet.

Evidence indicates that it can go a long way to minimize or even avoid thyroid disorders by consuming a diet rich in unique nutrients. When you look at just what those nutrients are, it's obvious to see that most of them are in meat.

In particular, zinc can stimulate thyroid hormones in hypothyroidism and is not in short supply from a diet rich in beef. All meats are, in truth, recommended for those who need to increase the development of thyroid hormone. It's also worth noting that it has been shown that weight loss on a low-carb diet helps reduce the development of excess thyroid hormones. That implies that increased intake of meat will enhance this situation all around.

1.6 Side Effects of carnivore diet and their Cures?

Without its health consequences, no diet appears that's also part of the carnivore diet. Fortunately, on an animal-based diet, the human body performs exceptionally well, and any harmful side effects are temporary. Here are a few side effects of a carnivorous diet and how to treat them.

DIARRHEA ON CARNIVORE DIET

Your gastrointestinal tract may experience disruptions if you have diarrhea, feel uneasy in the bathroom, or get alarming signals from the digestive system.

What happens?

Diarrhea may happen when food moves too rapidly through your digestive tract. Transit times are typically slower if you've been consuming plant foods to give your body time to cope with the extra fiber and extract nutrients from the food. Transit time can be affected as you move to a zero-fiber diet and diarrhea occurs.

What's the effective cure?

On the carnivore diet, the treatment for diarrhea is:

Give your body time to adjust to a zero-fiber diet - food can move too quickly through the large intestine at first so that the large intestine pulls water from the food.

Minimize the intake of rendered fats - liquid fats such as tallow and cream are commonly rendered fats. These fat types can move too easily through your system.

BAD BREATH ON THE CARNIVORE DIET

One of the side effects of going from a high protein diet using glucose as the primary fuel source to a low carb diet while using ketones as a fuel source is bad breath. "The "keto breath" is often considered to.

What Happens?

Compound acetone is responsible for the change in the scent of your breath. Acetone is the simplest and perhaps most rapidly changing of the various forms of ketones and is formed from acetoacetate, ketone muscle dissolution. Acetone disperses into the lungs during ketosis and leaves the body as you exhale.

What's the effective cure?

Some individuals don't get a keto breath, but with time, it goes away on its own for those who do. If you do have it, during the carnivore diet, there are some things you can do to minimize bad breath.

Wait - if it's not that bad, sitting it out and waiting for it to go on its own is OK.

Drink more - As you urinate, ketones can often leave the body, so drinking more water will also eliminate extra ketones in the urine.

Stay fresh- Keep your teeth, tongue, gums, and mouth clean so the air you breathe does not mix with any other unpleasant odors.

HEART PALPITATIONS ON THE CARNIVORE DIET

The carnivore diet's common symptom is heart palpitations, beating heart, and flutters, but it is generally episodic and nothing to stress about in these situations.

What Happens

It's normal to find that your heart rate increases, or your stroke volume increases when you first adopt a carnivore diet. It is generally due to a lower blood volume, dehydration, and a loss of electrolytes, which can be the product of low blood volume. The heart needs to toughen up to work harder to maintain the blood pressure when you feel those fast heartbeats.

What's the effective cure?

Drinking enough water is the easiest cure and ensuring that you keep the salt your body requires will help fight those palpitations in the heart. Additional options include:

Take some magnesium - the recommended daily amount is up to 400 mg per day and is safe for most individuals.

Get on point with your salt intake - too little or too much can cause palpitations in the chest. It's probably more likely that you have too little rather than too many.

Add in carbs - You will need to add more carbs to raise blood flow if the heart palpitations do not go away within a few weeks.

HIGH CHOLESTEROL ON THE CARNIVORE DIET

What Happens?

The Carnivore Diet is high in sodium, cholesterol and fat, and the elevation of your cholesterol levels may be one of the diet's most important concerns. The rise in saturated fat increases your levels of cholesterol with time. Cholesterol, however, is not bad. The media and recent studies show that low carb and higher fat diets can contribute to an improved lipid profile.

What's the effective cure?

Before you start the carnivore diet, have your cholesterol levels tested first and foremost, so you have a baseline on which to operate. There are a few things you can do if you get a relevant lipid profile on the carnivore diet:

Reduce the consumption of liquid fat. It can also, on its own, boost your lipid profile.

For at least 12 hours a day, try fasting. There is sufficient evidence to suggest that this would lower total cholesterol levels.

Consult the physician. Most doctors are willing to speak with you about your carnivore way of life and give suggestions, particularly younger ones.

LEG CRAMPS ON CARNIVORE DIET

Among those who just started the carnivore diet, leg cramps are a frequent issue, but they typically fade over time. With that said, on the carnivore diet, there are some items you can do to avoid or remove leg cramps completely.

What Happens?

Muscle cramps are caused by the change of nutrients, especially magnesium. Consequently, it is also not unusual to get leg cramps due to low potassium or sodium intake.

What's the effective cure?

On the carnivore diet, leg cramps treatment is to even magnesium, sodium, and potassium levels. It can attain in two ways:

Increase sodium - Maybe the best way to balance your mineral levels is to add additional salt to your diet to avoid mineral loss. As levels of sodium decline, amounts of magnesium and potassium normally follow.

Supplement - consider replacing with magnesium in some situations where more sodium does not help.

Slow down - you might want some more time to adapt and in the worst situation where nothing works. Although pushing through is possible, it's also OK to add more carbs and then slowly decrease them over time to allow your body time to adjust.

Adaption: Nausea, Headaches, Lack of focus, Irritability

Due to your body's normal reaction to carbohydrate limitation and the elimination of unnecessary chemicals and additives, you will notice some unpleasant side effects and side symptoms during adaptation.

Some of the other effects of the adaption process include headache, chills, digestive issues, dizziness, irritability, bad breath/smell, dry mouth, brain fog, nausea, bad taste in the mouth, poor focus, insomnia, decreased physical performance, sore throat cramping, cravings, diarrhea, rapid heart rate, night sweats, poor focus, and muscle soreness.

These effects are the result of significant hormonal and metabolic changes.

What Happens?

Your body will have to re-learn about using fat as a source of energy as the muscle glycogen levels start dropping due to a lack of carbohydrate intake. It takes time for this "switch," and you feel low energy during that time, feel irritable and extreme cravings. How much you suffer will depend on how metabolically active you are.

As if that weren't enough, while your gallbladder and pancreas react to the extra fat intake, you may also notice gastrointestinal problems such as diarrhea.

Finally, the hormones will take a hit as your body re-balances minerals, fluids, and sources of energy. T3 and Cortisol, in particular. T3 is a thyroid hormone that depends on carbohydrates' ingestion to manage metabolism, and Cortisol would be a stress hormone.

What's the effective cure?

Many of the signs of adjusting to the carnivore diet can be minimized or even removed using a couple of easy tricks:

Eat more - the carnivore diet is naturally full of protein and high in fat, ensuring you can feel satisfied for a very long time. It could mean your daily intake of calories is much smaller. Find out how many calories you have to live and then consider when deciding on the amount of food.

Drink more - it's natural to drop a lot of fluids, particularly during the first few days, but if you don't want to experience the symptoms, these fluids need to be replaced.

Electrolytes - you can need more electrolytes if more water and food don't help. First, try to add some extra salt to your diet, but suggest an electrolyte supplement if you need to.

Sweat more - exercise is a perfect way to naturally eliminate excess contaminants and re-equalize the electrolyte levels.

Chapter 2: Breakfast Recipes for the Carnivore Diet

You may not have eaten for up to 10 hours when you wake up after your overnight sleep. Breakfast recharges the body's energy and nutrient reserves. In a brief period, it increases the energy levels and ability to focus and can decrease the risk of type 2 diabetes, long-term heart disease and improved weight management.

75. 1. Carnivore Breakfast Sandwich

It's delicious, easy, and rich in protein, fat, with no plants. This breakfast sandwich is appreciated by those on the carnivore diet or anyone who loves their diet with fat and protein. Although the Carnivore Breakfast Sandwich appears to criticize the mainstream cholesterol-preventing dietary advice, what we enjoy about this breakfast sandwich is how Incredibly delicious it is!

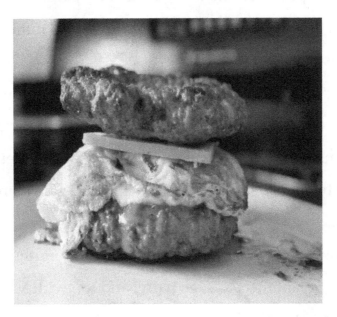

Prep Time: 5 Minutes

Cook Time: 5 Minutes

Total Time: 10 Minutes

Serving: 1

INGREDIENTS

- One egg

- One tsp bacon grease or butter.

- Two Sausage Patties beef

- 1-ounce cheddar cheese

INSTRUCTIONS

1. Melt butter on moderate temperature in a big skillet.

2. Shape the sausage into thin patties, about 1/2 inch thick but about the length of the palm. On the other side, cook patties until it turns to brown color, then flip, cook the other side for further 2-3 minutes, till then cooking continuously.

3. Fry an egg in the same pan at the same time. If not, in an additional pan (moderate temperature and take some time until the pan is hot to avoid sticking), use a little more butter and then prepare your carnivore breakfast sandwich. As with your sauce and keep sauce thin with yolk.

4. Set one sausage patty on a tray for preparation, then top it with a slice of cheese egg, another sausage patty, and top with a fried egg.

5. You can add sliced onion, sautéed spinach, or avocado as well. Enjoy the meal.

76. 2. Cheesy 3-Meat Breakfast Casserole Recipe

There's all in this Cheesy 3-Meat Breakfast Casserole recipe: sausage, plenty of cheese, bacon, and ham. Perfect for a weekend breakfast or even during the holidays for visitors. A breakfast for lovers of meat!

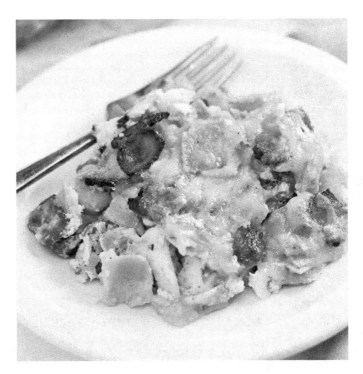

Prep Time: 15 Minutes

Cook Time: 40 Minutes

Total Time: 55 Minutes

Servings: 10

Ingredients

- Seven ounces of ham chopped.

- Potatoes cut into cubes.

- 32 ounces chilled hash brown

- Two cups shredded cheddar cheese.

- Two cups of milk, eight large eggs, one tsp of salt.

- One medium onion (diced)

- Half teaspoon pepper.

- Twelve ounces breakfast sausage

- Twelve ounces bacon (diced into 1" pieces)

- Half tsp. garlic powder

Instructions

1. Spray with cooking spray on a 9x13" baking dish. Preheat oven to 350°F.

2. Cook the bacon pieces in a large non - stick frying pan once cooked thoroughly and become crispy. Don't overcook anymore. Remove the bacon from the bowl with a slotted spoon, leave the grease in the pan. Cook the sausage in the same frying pan over medium-high heat, breaking up the connections so that you have bite-sized bits (or smaller). When the sausage is roughly halfway finished, add the onion, and cook until the sausage is fully cooked. Stir the sausage/onion mixture into a bowl with a slotted spoon and leave the pan's grease.

3. After cooking both the bacon and the sausage and removing them from the pan, add the pan's brown hash potatoes. Cook the potatoes in the remaining grease over medium heat until they are softened and

browned slightly. In the lower part of the prepared baking dish, layer the hash browns.

4. Layer the cooked bacon on top of the hash browns, the ham, and the sausage/onion mixture. Then, scatter the cheese equally over the beef.

5. Whisk the eggs with the milk, garlic powder, salt, and pepper together in a big cup. On the upper side of the covered ingredients of the baking dish, add the egg mixture on top.

6. Bake for about 35-40 minutes in the oven or until the egg is fully set and the cheese is soft and bubbly.

77. 3. One-Pan Egg and Turkey Skillet Recipe

You now need to have this One-Pan Egg and Turkey Skillet if you are looking for an easy, nutritious, and delicious meal. You're going to love that. The most important meal of the day is breakfast. So, with this balanced breakfast, start your day right off.

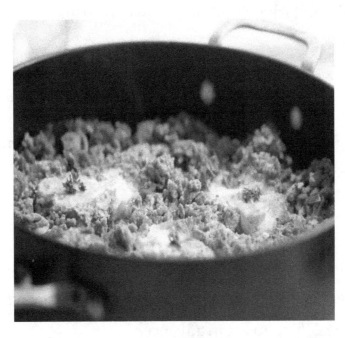

Prep Time: 5 Minutes

Cook Time: 20 Minutes

Total Time: 25 Minutes

Servings: 6

INGREDIENTS

- Six eggs

- One cup salsa

- Pepper and salt according to taste.

- 1 pound ground turkey

INSTRUCTIONS

1. Spray with non-stick cooking spray on the skillet and add in ground turkey.

2. Cook until the turkey is golden brown, over moderate flame. Also, drain all grease.

3. Connect the salsa mixture and blend well. For 2-3 minutes, cook the turkey and salsa.

4. Put the eggs in the skillet and cover them for 7 to 9 minutes or until the eggs are cooked to your taste.

78. 4. Keto and Carnivore Meatloaf Muffin

It's quick to make this amazing Keto and Carnivore Meatloaf Muffin Meal, tasty but without all the fillers and perfect for taking for work or breakfast on-the-go. You can keep them all week long to eat in advance.

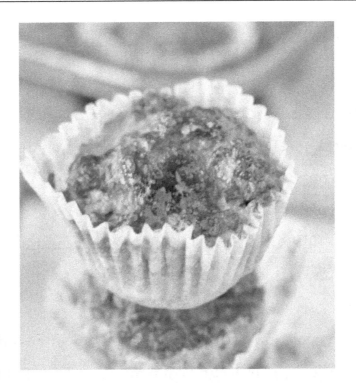

Prep Time: 15 Minutes

Cook Time: 25 Minutes

Servings: 2

Ingredients

- Two eggs

- 2 lbs. 85 percent ground beef

- Two tsps. Sea salt.

Optional Ingredients:

- Two tsps. paprika

- No-sugar added ketchup for topping.

- One tbsp. garlic powder

- Half tsp. black powder

Instructions

1. To 350 degrees, set the oven.

2. Mix the eggs, meat, spices, and salt, if used, in a large mixing bowl with both hands until well mixed.

3. Using the liners to prepare the muffin pan.

4. Use meat to fill each cup until it is three times the amount filled.

5. Put the muffins in the oven with the meatloaf and put it in the oven for 25-35 minutes.

6. Muffins can cook quicker or slower, based on your oven.

7. Check a muffin by gently cut the hot muffin in half after about 20 minutes.

8. Take the muffin pan from the oven. If it seems done enough in your taste, present the muffins with tongs, and eat.

79. 5. Carnivore Keto Burgers

If you are considering the Carnivore diet, these burgers will become one of your favorite meals. You get enough calories from this to keep your energy up, so fattier meat cuts are best.

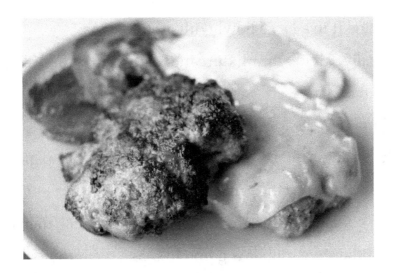

Prep Time: 5 Minutes

Cook Time: 10 Minutes

Total Time: 15 Minutes

Servings: 8

Ingredients

- One teaspoon salt.

- 200 grams Speck or bacon 0.5 pound

- 500 grams Ground Beef (Beef grind) 1 pound

- 500 grams Ground Pork (Pork grind) 1 pound

- Two tablespoons Southwest Seasoning

Instructions

1. Cut the speck to the smallest possible size. If you want everything chopped/ground more equally, you can also use a mincer or food processor.

2. Combine it in a large bowl with all the items.

3. Generally, divide the mixture into eight patties and shape each by hand into a patty style.

4. BBQ on high/heat grill

5. Switch the grill/Barbeque down to low and put patties and straighten with a spatula on the grill/BBQ.

6. Please enable it to cook for 5 minutes on the grill, then flipped and cook for another five min. It is going to make the burgers well done.

7. Add and display your favorite seasonings.

80. 6 Low-carb baked eggs

A great low-carb combination of eggs and beef. Please, yes! At any moment, cook up this delicious gem-lunch, dinner, or breakfast. You will be thanked by your every taste buds!

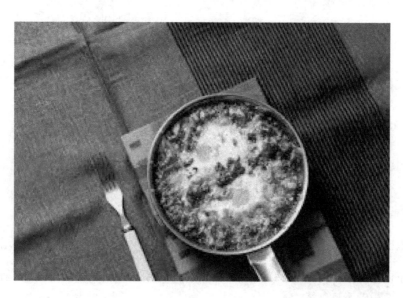

Prep Time: 5 Minutes

Cook Time: 10 Minutes.

Serving: 1

Ingredients

- Two eggs

- Half cup (2 oz.) grated cheese

- Three oz. Ground turkey or ground pork or ground beef cook it any way you like.

Instructions

1. Heat the oven to 200 °C (400 °F).
2. Arrange a cooked mixture of ground beef in a little baking dish. Then, using a spoon, make two holes and crack the eggs into them.
3. Sprinkle the end with shredded cheese.
4. Cook in the oven for around 10-15 minutes, till the eggs are cooked.
5. Allow it to cool for a little while. The ground meat and eggs get very hot.

Tip for the recipe

- It is a great recipe for the remaining hamburger you weren't sure what to do. Accumulate the recipe by the number of people and the entire family; you'll have dinner. Tada!

- Complement this with fresh herbs and avocado with quite a crunchy, crisp salad. Or give this a try with this amazing homemade mayonnaise (made without additives and soybean oil).

81. 7. Spam and Eggs

A delicious recipe eaten for lunch, breakfast, or dinner is this easy Spam and Eggs. These cheesy meat eggs in less than fifteen min make a perfect, fast breakfast!

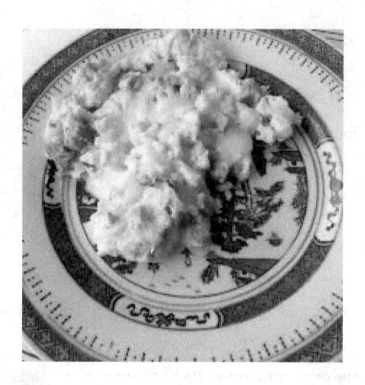

Prep Time: 5 Minutes.

Cook Time: 10 Minutes.

Total Time: 15 Minutes

Servings: 2

Ingredients

- Two eggs are well beaten.

- Two ounces Cheddar cheese, shredded.

- One (12 ounces) bowl of fully cooked luncheon meat (for example, spam) cut into cubes.

Instructions

Under moderate heat on a non-stick pan, put the eggs in, then spam. Cooked and stir till the eggs are almost ready, then spread over the cheese and mix until it is melted.

Chapter 3: Lunch Recipes for Carnivore Diet

The lunch hour helps your brain to relax, refresh, and remain focused, although it will directly increase your productivity for the rest of the day. Taking some time out during the day, yet if you choose to take some brief breaks, offers your brain an opportunity to recharge. Getting the proper ratio of meals is the secret to a balanced packed lunch to give you the nutrition you have to remain healthy.

82. 1. Carnivore Chicken Nuggets

Everyone enjoys chicken nuggets. This beautiful and tasty recipe is simple and full of nutrients to develop. Appreciate the meals which everyone enjoys in a healthily!

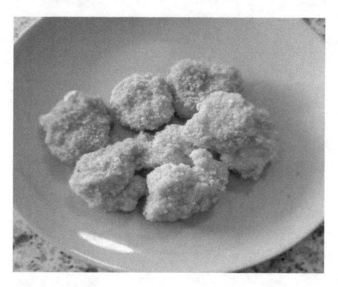

Prep Time: 40 minutes

Cook Time: 20 minutes

Servings: 60 nuggets.

Ingredients

- One large egg

- Mixture of bread

- half teaspoon oregano

- One cup of parmesan cheese is shredded.

- One cup pork rinds ground

- Three lbs. ground chicken or chop your own.

- Chicken Mixture

- half teaspoon pink salt

Instructions

1. Preheat the oven to 400°C.

2. Step cookie sheet with baking paper.

3. In a flat pan, merge the cheese and ground pork.

4. Stir up your egg, spices, and chicken.

5. From the chicken mixture, shape a small patty of the size you want. On the breading, put the mixture.

6. Cover the chicken with the mixture using a fork.

7. Place it on a cookie sheet lined with parchment.

8. Please continue with steps 5 - 7 till you have used all the chicken. If you are out of bread, make more of it.

9. Bake for 20 minutes at 400 degrees.

83. 2. Cheesy Air Fryer Meatballs

You can make tasty, healthy meatballs in even less than thirty min, without any greasy mess! Real easy low carb meal in your air fryer for Cheesy Meatballs made fast and easy. Perfect for those who are on the carnivore diet.

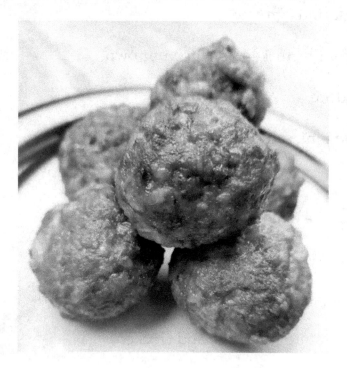

Prep Time: 20 Minutes

Cook Time: 12 Minutes

Resting Time: 8 Minutes

Total Time: 40 Minutes

Servings: 6 (4 meat-balls servings)

Equipment

Air Fryer

Ingredients

- One tablespoon lard

- 2 ounces pork rinds

- Three ounces shredded Italian cheese blend.

- One teaspoon pink sea salt

- Two pounds grass-fed ground beef

- Two large, well-blended eggs

Instructions

1. In a mixing bowl, add all of the items. Mash the mixture with clean hands till it is fully mixed.

2. Roll around 1 1/2 inches in diameter into balls. Twenty-four meatballs will be prepared by this method.

3. You'll cook them in parts, which vary according to the size of your air fryer.

4. If you use them, fill your fryer basket with liners. Otherwise, spray with cooking spray.

5. Put meatballs in the basket, ensuring they do not touch the basket's sides and each other.

6. Cook for 8 minutes at 350 degrees. Bring the basket out and switch over the balls of meat. Return to the frying pan and cook for another 4 minutes at 350 degrees.

7. The core temperature of the meatballs should approach 165 degrees, and then they're cooked!

84. 3. Scallops with Wrapped Bacon

Jumbo scallops covered in a flavorful glaze are the bacon-wrapped scallops and broiled to satisfaction. A quick but tasteful appetizer and the main course choice that will get rave reviews for sure!

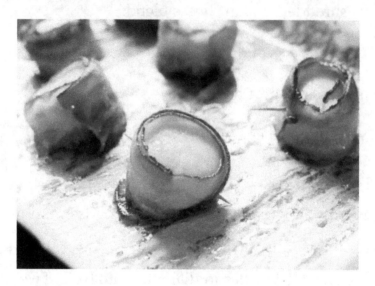

Prep Time: 20 minutes

Cook Time: 15 minutes

Total Time: 35 minutes

Servings: 6

INGREDIENTS

- One-pound bacon slices diced in the half crossway.

- Two tablespoons of well-diced parsley.

- Two tablespoons soy sauce

- Pepper and salt according to your taste.

- 2 pounds large sea scallops patted dry.

- A cup of quarter fourth maple syrup

- 1/4 teaspoon garlic powder and

- cooking spray

INSTRUCTIONS

1. Preheat your broiler. Utilizing cooking spray to cover a sheet pan.

2. Cover each scallop around a slice of bacon and fix it with a toothpick. Put the scallops on the baking pan in a single layer.

3. Whisk all together soy sauce, pepper, salt, garlic powder and maple syrup in a small cup. Brush from over the top from each of the scallops with half the paste.

4. Broil around 10-15 minutes, just until the bacon becomes crispy and cooked through scallops. Half the way through the cooking process, brush the leftover sauce and over scallops.

5. Sprinkle parsley and serve.

85. 4. Steak Tartare

If you are on the carnivore diet and love healthy, fresh flavors, this homemade Steak Tartare (or Beef Tartare) is something you can make at home.

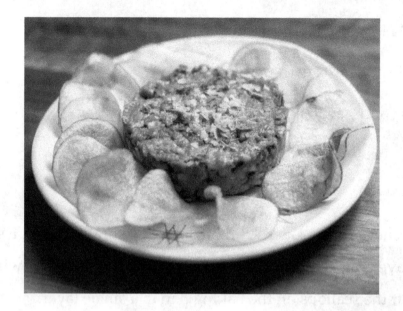

Total Time: 30 minutes (includes freezing time)

Active Time: 25 minutes

Servings: 4

Ingredients:

- Two large egg yolks

- Six tbsps. finely diced shallots

- One tsp. kosher salt

- Half tsp. dry mustard

- Two tsps. sherry vinegar

- Sixteen ounces top sirloin cleaned and trimmed.

- 2 tbsps. Fresh parsley is finely diced and divided.

- One tsp. freshly grated lemon zest

- 1/4 cup celery leaves are finely diced and divided.

- 1/4 cup light olive oil

- Two tbsps. Small brined capers drained and unrinsed.

Instructions

1. Custom instruments: pastry ring 3 3/4-inch, food processor (optional)

2. Slice the steak into 1-inch pieces and set aside for 10 mins in the refrigerator.

3. In a small bowl, mix dry mustard, egg yolks, and vinegar. Stir continuously until caramelized while streaming in the oil, then whisk in the salt, shallots, capers, parsley, and around 2/3 of the celery leaves.

4. Cut the meat to your preferred shape through the hand. (Likewise, distribute the meat in 4 quantities and pulse each batch in the food processor bowl fitted with the regular S-blade 3 to 4 times separately.)

5. With neat hands, bend the meat and flavor it easily. Plate and garnish with the lemon zest and reserved herbs using a 3 3/4-inch pastry ring.

86. 5. Low-Carb Beef Bourguignon Stew

It is likely to obtain this dish of Low-Carb Beef Bourguignon Stew in an Instant Pot or slow cooker. It can be enjoyed by those on Atkins, low carb, keto, diabetics, gluten-free, Paleo, grain-free, or Banting Diet.

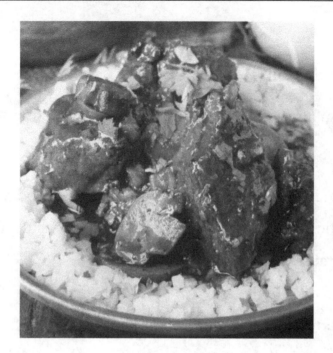

Prep Time: 30 minutes

Cook Time: 30 minutes

Total Time: 1 hour

Servings: 6

Ingredients

- Four ounces white onion (about 1 small)

- Two stalks celery sliced.

- Eight ounces of mushrooms thickly cut into pieces.

- 1 1/2-pound stew meat diced into 1 1/2 -2-inch cubes and dry with a paper towel.

- Four pieces of bacon cut crosswise.

- 1/4 tsp. Black pepper freshly ground.

- 1/2 tsp. sea salt (or to taste)

- 1 cup dry burgundy wine

- 1/2 tsp. dried thyme

- 1 tbsp. Fresh parsley chopped.

- One clove of garlic crushed.

- Half tsp. Xanthan gum.

- One cup beef stock or, you can use low-salt broth.

- Two tbsps. tomato paste

- One bay leaf

Instructions

Instant Pot instructions

1. As the Instant Pot covers off, select the sauté mode. Add the bacon when the "hot" sign appears. Cook the bacon till crispy, mixing frequently. Remove it to a plate lined with paper towels. Do not remove grease comprising bacon.

2. To an Instant Kettle, add half of the beef. Use the pepper and salt to sprinkle. Before flipping, make the first side brown. Brown both ends of it and pull it to a tray. For the other half of the beef, repeat. If during this process, the Instant Pot switches off, set again to Sauté.

3. Discharge of all but one tablespoon of the pot's drippings. (Add around a tablespoon of recommended oil or butter to the Instant

Pot if there is less than one tablespoon) Continue with the sauté setting and add the celery and onion to the pot. Please enable it to cook until it starts to soften. Add the mushrooms. Cook the vegetables until they begin to soften the mushrooms. Stir in the garlic and cook for a moment. Transfer to a dish.

4. Add about a teaspoon if there's no oil left in the pot. To the pot, add the xanthan gum. Stir through the xanthan gum to spread the oil. Pour the burgundy in and mix, scraping the brown pieces together. Simmer until the wine begins to thicken. Add broth of beef. Whisk in the tomato paste, thyme, and bay leaf. Just take it to a simmer. Enable to boil until the broth thickens enough for a spoon to stick. Send browned chunks of beef (including the drippings) and bacon to the pot of vegetables. Stir in the salt and pepper.

5. Cover Instant Pot. "Steam release location handle for "Sealing." To change the time to 30 minutes, select the Meat/Stew feature and press the +/- button. Used this Quick Release method (follow Instant Pot instruction book) to vent the Instant Pot when the stew is finished. Press Cancel. When opening the lid, be sure the float valve is down.

6. Taste the seasoning and adjust. Until serving, cut the bay leaf and sprinkle it with parsley.

Slow cooker instructions:

(add 5 hours and 30 minutes to cooking time)

1. On moderate flame, heat the Dutch oven or large soup pot. Add the bacon when the pot is hot. Cook the bacon till crisp, stirring occasionally. Lift to a plate lined with paper towels to clean and transfer to the slow cooker.

2. To the pot, put 1/2 of the beef. Chunks shouldn't harm you. Using pepper and salt to sprinkle. Before flipping, cause the first side to brown. Then brown flip both sides to the slow cooker. For the other part of the meat, return.

3. Discharge of all but 1 tbsp of the pot's drippings. If less than a tablespoon is available, add a little of the oil of your choice. Cl Continue to add the celery and onions to the pot over moderate temperature. Please enable it to cook till it starts to soften. Add the mushrooms. Cook the vegetables until they begin to soften the mushrooms. Stir in the garlic and boil for a minute. Place the vegetables in a crockpot.

4. Add about a teaspoon of your oil choice if there is no oil left in the tank. To the jar, add the xanthan gum. Stir in the oil to spread it. Pour the burgundy in and stir, scraping the brown bits together. Simmer and simmer until the wine begins to thicken. Add broth of beef. Stir in the tomato paste, bay leaf, and thyme. Just bring it to a simmer. Enable to boil until the broth thickens enough for a spoon to coat. Stir in the pepper and salt. Shift the bacon, beef, and vegetables to the slow cooker and mix.

5. Then seal the slow cooker. Process the stew for six-eight hours or until meat is cooked.

6. Taste and change the seasoning when served. Before serving, extract the bay leaf and sprinkle it with parsley.

87. 6. Lunch Meat Roll-Ups

Lunch Meat Roll-Ups seem to be simple to create, adaptable enough to suit everyone's different interests, and make an ideal keto lunch or healthy meal! As specific and over the edge as you prefer, you can also make these roll-ups!

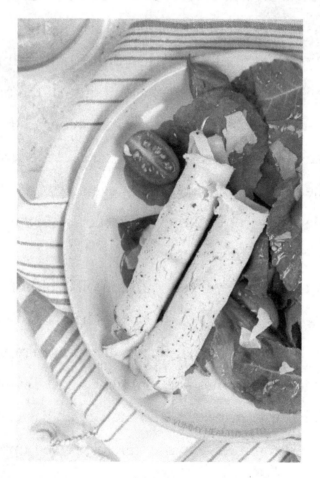

Prep Time: 5 minutes

Total Time: 5 minutes

Servings: 2

Ingredients

- Four pieces of cheese

- Four pieces of lunch meat

- garnishes of your preference if you want shredded lettuce, herb cream cheese, guacamole.

- black pepper and sea salt

Instructions

1. On the workplace surface, put your meat pieces and garnish them with a cheese slice.

2. Note: This would be a wonderful time to guacamole or dressings of your choice on top, herb spread cream cheese,

3. Wrap your lunch meat across the cheese till you have a log, starting from the bottom.

4. Continue to roll up your rolls of meat and cheese until you reach the amount you would like. Use black pepper and sea salt to sprinkle.

5. Serve with a leafy green salad or bowl of bone broth.

Note

Please press on your lunch meat's thicker side to be cut to be smoother to roll and remain together.

7. Carnivore Braised Beef Shank

It's a highly versatile recipe that can be made from a cast-iron skillet or Dutch oven to a crockpot to an instant pot with multiple cooking equipment. You can also slow-cook it in the oven rather than cooking on the stovetop. You get a delicious lunchtime recipe!

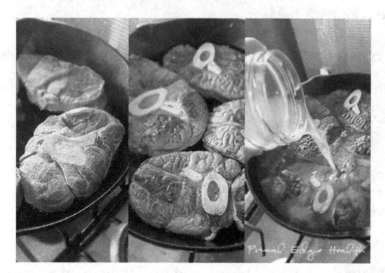

Prep Time: 5 Minutes

Cook Time: 3 hrs.

Total Time: 3 hrs. 5 mins

Servings: 4

EQUIPMENT

Cast iron skillet.

Dutch oven

INGREDIENTS

- Two-three cups of bone broth or water

- One tbsp ghee, beef tallow butter or other cooking fat.

- Four pieces beef shank 1-inch thick, eight ounces each

- One tsp. Salt or as you required.

INSTRUCTIONS

1. In the Dutch oven or cast iron or heavy bottom skillet with cover, burn the cooking fat. Brown from both sides of the beef shanks till a golden-brown crust forms, about 2-3 minutes each side.

2. Over shanks, pour the broth. Use 2 cups of broth, at least. The considerable broth will be acceptable 1/2 to 3/4 of the way up the side to cover the meat, with salt, season. Bring a boil to it.

3. Reduce heat and cover the pot and let the steam escape from a tiny hole.

4. Cook for 3 hours, over a low flame, till the meat begins to fall off the bone. Serve warm in liquid.

NOTES

- Over the last 30 minutes of the cooking process, add any of the vegetables and herbs mentioned above and cook with the meat.

- Oven method Follow steps 1-2, then place the lid on after broth is simmering and switch to the oven for 2 hours for the roast.

- Crockpot Method put meat in a slow cooker's bottom, pour broth over and sprinkle with salt. Cover it with your cover and turn it down. Cooked for 4-6 hours before the bone breaks down easily.

- Seasoning the meat with the instant pot method. Turn the Instant pot on and choose to sauté. When heated, add the cooking fat to the pot and cook the meat until golden brown, around 2-3 minutes on each side. Add some broth. Close the sealing valve and lid. Put the high pressure in order and cook for 35 minutes. For 15 minutes, the normal release pressure releases the remaining pressure gradually.

88. 8. Herb Roasted Bone Marrow

Marrow is an outstanding substitute of the omega-3s essential for safe brain growth and anti-inflammation. It's very, very beneficial for everyone.

It's fairly affordable if you prepare it straight away (versus having it at a fine dining restaurant). It's incredibly tasty.

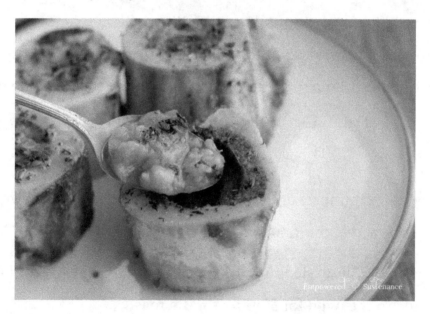

Prep time: 5 mins

Cook time: 15 mins.

Total time: 20 mins

Servings: 1-2 marrow bones

INGREDIENTS

- Fresh rosemary

- Marrow bones from grass-fed/pasture-raised beef, 1-2 each person

- black pepper and salt

- Fresh thyme

INSTRUCTIONS

1. For one person, the marrow with one or two pieces of bone is quite enough.

2. Defrost it properly if the bones are frozen.

3. To 400 degrees, set the oven. In a baking dish, put the bones. Spacing does not matter - closely or loosely, it is spaced.

4. Finely chop the thyme and fresh rosemary into equal parts. Use 1/2 teaspoon of chopped herbs for four marrow bones. Over the marrow bones, sprinkle the spices.

5. Roast for around fifteen min, until the inside is no longer pink. Until the marrow starts to "cook out" of the bones, you had to catch them.

6. Serve hot and season with salt and pepper. Scoop out the marrow using a spoon.

7. Save any drippings in an airtight jar in the refrigerator for a few days, as well as the remaining marrow. Chop the leftover marrow finely and toss it for a flavor and nutrient boost with hot, cooked vegetables.

Chapter 4: Desserts and Snack Recipes for the Carnivore Diet

After all, it's all about satisfying the soul with food for dessert enthusiasts that allows them to realize like they've reached Paradise on earth at last. Eating dessert does not indicate that you have little or no control over yourself. It just means you've got a clear idea of what you want (it's just a delicious blueberry cheesecake sometimes), and you've got what it takes to satisfy these cravings.

89. 1. Bacony Carnivore Womelletes

This one is excellent topped with cinnamon butter as well as a pour of pancake syrup without sugar. For sandwiches, it also stands up very well.

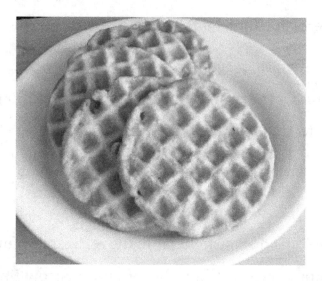

Prep Time: 2 minutes

Cook Time: 8 minutes

Total Time: 10 minutes

Servings: 2 womelletes.

INGREDIENTS

- One large egg.

- One slice of bacon (raw)

- hefty pinch of any spices or flavorings as you want.

- Splash maple extract, if required.

INSTRUCTIONS

1. Put the bacon in a food processor or blender and turn it on.

2. Put any seasonings and egg down the chute until the bacon is ground up and start operating the machine till liquified and well-in incorporated. It is your womelletes slurry.

3. As per its directions, warm your mini-waffle machine.

4. In a waffle maker, add half the slurry and place the cover around.

5. Cook for around 3-5 mins max till golden or to your preferred level of flavor and texture.

6. Take away from the waffle maker, and with the leftover slurry, repeat the procedure 4 and 5.

7. Enjoy the womelletes warm or as you are delighted.

90. 2. Carnivore Cake

While you follow the carnivore diet strictly and sometimes seem to desire a dessert, well, we have nothing sweet for you, but we've got a cake.

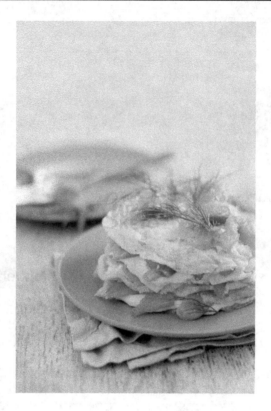

Prep Time: 5 minutes

Cook Time: 10 minutes

Total Time: 25 minutes

Servings: 8

INGREDIENTS

- Seven oz creamy cheese

- One pinch of dill for decoration

- Ten oz smoked salmon

- Eight eggs

- One pinch salt

INSTRUCTIONS

1. Inside a small bowl, beat the salt and eggs until mixed.

2. Heat skillet or 6-in nonstick pan over the moderate flame while heated.

3. To coat the pan's base, pour 1/4 cup of the mixture into the pan and whisk. Adjust the pan to the flame and allow the eggs to cook.

4. Cooked the egg crepes till they are just set (about 30 seconds) on the bottom, so there is no browning on the sides. Turn gently over the crepe and cook on the opposite side for a couple of seconds.

5. Repeat till all the mixture is used.

6. To cool off, place the cooking crepes on a wire rack or a plate.

Let us bring everything together.

- Bring one crepe upon this plate and cover it with a thin coating of cream cheese.

- Layer cream cheese with diced smoked salmon and top with next crepe.

- Continue layering till all components are being used.

- Customize and serve with dill.

NOTE:

In the refrigerator, let the cake stay for 1 hour; it'll be smoother to break. For decorative purposes, utilize fresh dill.

3. Egg Custard

With its elegant yet mild taste and its creaminess, this traditional dessert is still a highlight. Preferably sized for a children's treat yet mature enough for a formal dinner, it requires just 15 minutes to prepare and can be kept for up to 3 days in the fridge, sealed. (The evening once you've made this is much better.)

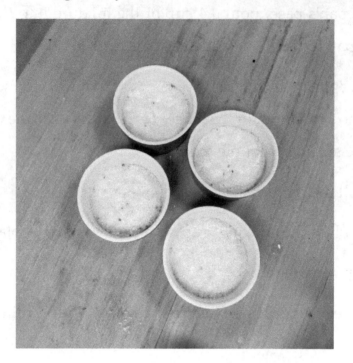

Prep Time: 10 minutes

Cook Time: 2 hours.

Servings: 6

INGREDIENTS

- Two eggs

- Two cups whole milk

- Two egg yolks

- 1/3 cup sugar

- Freshly shredded or ground nutmeg

- One tsp. of vanilla extract

PREPARATION

1. Heat the oven around 300 degrees.

2. Placed in a deep baking pan broad enough to accommodate six 4-ounce ovenproof cups (you can use coffee cups or ramekins marked as oven-safe).

3. Get the milk to a boil with moderate flame in a medium-size saucepan.

4. In the meantime, mix the yolks, sugar, vanilla, and eggs in a distinct dish.

5. Through boiling milk, stir the egg mixture, stirring gently to incorporate.

6. Pour the mixture into the cups via a fine strainer (unless the strainer clogs, choose a spoon to scrape it clean), then drizzled with the nutmeg gently.

7. In the pan, pour hot (not boiling) water till it hits half the way up the cups' ends.

8. Bake for 30 to 35 minutes until the custard is just finished (it can still be a bit loose).

9. Before served, just let the custard cool in cold water for around 2 hours.

4. Carnivore Chaffle Recipe

Because of the sauce, this meal has only one net carb. With a small salad aside, it can be served. It is very satisfying and tastes delicious! 1 serving in the oven renders this recipe.

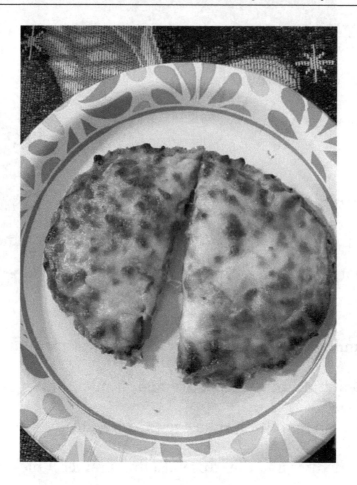

Prep Time: 3 minutes

Cook Time: 8 minutes

Serving: 1

INGREDIENTS

- 1/4 cup parmesan cheese shredded.

- 1/4 cup chopped pork rinds.

- One egg is well beaten.

- One tsp. Grill mate roasted garlic and herb flavoring.

INSTRUCTIONS

1. In a small bowl, mix all the ingredients and incorporate until thoroughly mixed.

2. Cover it with a silicone sheet or parchment paper using a small baking sheet.

3. Through wet hands, tap the mixture into a small circle or use a silicone spatula to create the pizza crust.

4. The oven baking duration is bake around each side for 10 minutes at 350 degrees in the oven.

5. Mini Dash Waffle Maker: Split the mixture into two and cook every other serving for at least 4 minutes before a crust forms (it could take longer if you are using a large waffle iron)

6. Air Fryer Baking Time: Cook on each side at 300 degrees for eight minutes.

7. If you prefer to remove the carnivore pizza crust with any seasonings and place the keto-friendly sauce of choice on. Mostly prefer black olives and Italian sausage.

8. Place 1/3 of mozzarella cheese on top.

9. Place the cheese in the oven, air fryer, or microwave until it becomes crispy, just long enough to melt. It takes just 1 minute for the microwave or 3 to 4 minutes for the oven or air fryer.

91. 5. Meat Bagels

A meat bagel is meat that has been molded into a bagel pattern and served like a bagel. For the keto, Paleo, low carb, and for those on the carnivore diet, it is the ideal bagel!

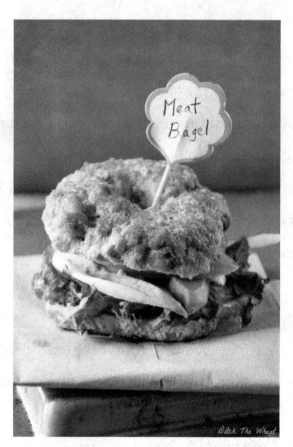

Prep Time: 15 minutes

Cook Time: 40 minutes

Total Time: 55 minutes

Serving: 6

INGREDIENTS

- Two pounds ground pork

- 2/3 cup of tomato sauce

- Two large eggs

- 1 ½ onion, finely diced.

- 1/2 tsp ground pepper

- One tablespoon butter/bacon/ grass-fed ghee fat etc.

- One teaspoon sea salt

- One teaspoon paprika

INSTRUCTIONS

1. Heat the oven to 400°F. Create a parchment paper baking dish.

2. Sauté the onions with some cooking fat over a moderate flame, like grass-fed ghee butter etc. Sauté once they're transparent. Before placing them in the meat, allow the onions to chill.

3. Adjust all the components in a dish, along with the fried onions. Blend enough to disperse the spices uniformly.

4. Distribute the meat into six pieces. Roll a piece into a ball utilizing the hands, shape the center, and straighten gently to create a bagel.

5. Put the meat-looking bagel in the dish and proceed with each of the meat parts.

6. Bake until the meat is completely cooked, or for 40 minutes.

7. Enable the cooling of the meat bagels. Just like a normal bagel, slice the meat bagel. Load the meat bagel with salads such as slices of onions, tomato, spinach, etc.

Chapter 5: Dinner Recipes for the Carnivore Diet

Dinner is also an essential meal, and with a variety of amazing foods, you can try new things. Better sleep, greater stress resilience, reduced inflammation, lower anxiety, improved digestion, and steady sugar levels are connected to a nutritious meal.

92. 1. Pot Roast Recipe with Gravy

Without lots of vegetables such as onions and garlic, you think you can't make Carnivore Diet Pot Roast because you are on the carnivore diet and can't consume vegetables. Here is the recipe, which is full of nutrition and quite easy to make.

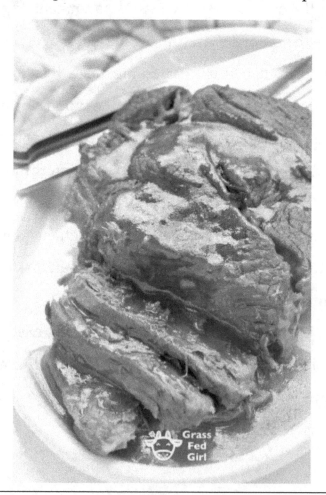

Prep Time: 10 minutes

Cook Time: 3 hours.

Servings: 4

Ingredients

- 1 4-5- lbs. pot roast

- Four tbsps. Butter or ghee.

- Two tsps. Sea salt.

- Three to Six cups of beef broth

Instructions

Recipe Notes

Cooking Time:

90 minutes Instant Pot

7 hours Slow Cooker

Stove Top

1. Heat the oven to 325°C. On both sides, salt the roast. On moderate temperature, heat the heavy bottom pan with a cover and put two tbsp of ghee.

2. Once the pan seems to be very hot, brown both sides of the roast from the surface for around 1-2 minutes.

3. From each side, whenever the pot roast is cooked, add the broth till the pot roast is coated and Put the cover and cook in the oven.

4. Bake in the oven for 2-3 hours, while enclosed, till it is fork-tender. Take it out of the oven and set off.

5. On moderate flame, place a small saucepan, add 1.5 cups of the remaining broth and the leftover 2 tbsp of ghee.

6. For 5-6 minutes, whisk the saucepan constantly till the broth decreases and thickens.

7. On a large dish, put the slice and roast crosswise. On over pot roast, put the thickened sauce.

8. Start serving and have a pleasant time.

Instant Pot

1. Turn on the device to sauté mode and dissolve the ghee.

2. For around two min each, add the pot roast and cook it on every side.

3. When the meat is wrapped, add the broth, and fix the cover, ensuring that the vent is covered.

4. Cooked for 90 minutes over high temperature.

5. Let the pressure automatically escape and ensure that it is a fork-tender.

6. Under moderate flame, put a small saucepan and pour 1.5 cups of the Instant Pot's remaining broth and two leftover tbsp of ghee.

7. For 5-6 mins, whisk the saucepan constantly till the broth decreases and thickens.

8. In the representing tray, move the pot roast and cut it crosswise.

9. Over the pot roast, spill the sauce. Start Serving and enjoy the meal.

Slow Cooker

1. Heat the frying pan on moderately high heat and dissolve the ghee.

2. Put the pot roast and cook it for about 2 minutes on every side till it is browned.

3. To the slow cooker, add the roast and add in the broth till it covers the meat.

4. About 6 hours, cooked on high heat as well as the meat is fork-tender.

5. Add 1.5 cups of broth and the leftover two tablespoons of ghee to a medium saucepan at moderate temperature.

6. For 3-5 minutes, stir the saucepan constantly until the broth decreases and thickens.

7. Move the pot roast to a serving dish and slice it crosswise into pieces.

8. On over pot roast, spill the thickened sauce. Present the meal and enjoy.

93. 2. Carnivore Skillet Pepperoni Pizza

A quick and simple Carnivore Skillet Pepperoni Pizza will fulfill the desire for pizza! Also, when you are on the Carnivore diet, no need to skip family pizza evening. One pan and just a couple of supplies!

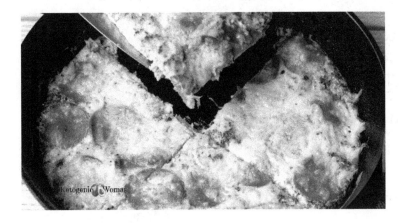

Prep Time: 10 Minutes

Cook Time: 15 Minutes

Total Time: 25 Minutes

Servings: 4

Ingredients

- 2 oz (1/2 cup) mozzarella cheese, grated.

- Four eggs.

- Pizza Base.

- Two tablespoon mayonnaise or melted butter, tallow, or lard.

- Pepperoni slices to cover the pizza.

- One tsp each garlic and onion powder.

- Pinch of salt for the taste.

- One teaspoon Italian seasoning.

- More Italian seasoning you can use if you need it.

- More cheese to sprinkle on top as you want it.

- Pizza Topping.

- 2 oz shredded parmesan.

Instructions

1. Heat the oven around 375°C.

2. Oil the cast iron frying pan.

3. Mix the cheese, eggs, seasoning and 2tbsp fat, all ingredients in a dish.

4. Into cast iron pan, add the mixture.

5. Sprinkle with some flavorings, cheese, and pepperoni on top.

6. Cook for 15 minutes in the oven or till the pizza is swollen and the layer starts to brown.

7. Slice it into four parts and try it!

3. Carnivore Ham and Cheese Noodle Soup

A Carnivore diet noodle recipe!? Cheese, bacon, bone broth, ham and fresh carnivore noodles are mixed in this rich cheesy, comforting nutritional soup! A pleasant change of style of the regular entry for the carnivore diet!

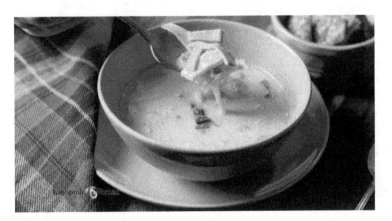

Prep Time: 15 Minutes

Cook Time: 15 Minutes

Total Time: 30 Minutes

Servings: 4

Ingredients

- 2 oz cream cheese cut into small pieces.

- 10-12 oz cubed cooked ham

- 1/4 cup bacon chopped or 3-4 pieces of cooked crisp bacon finely diced

- Two cups of bone broth or regular broth

- One cup Carnivore Noodles if you want it.

- Two cups cheddar cheese, shredded (save 1/2 cup for garnish)

- half cup heavy cream

- Pepper and Salt according to your taste.

Instructions

1. Heat the broth in a large medium pot until it almost begins to boil. Hold the broth at a reasonable volume.

2. Mix in the cubes of cream cheese and whisk until the broth is mixed and the chunks are removed.

3. Whisk in the finely chopped cheese till it mixes into the combination, about half a cup at a time.

4. Add the noodles and cubed ham and bring to a boil until fully cooked.

5. Mix in heavy cream and boil for a further min on low flame.

6. Cover each bowl with crumbled or chopped bacon and saved shredded cheddar cheese. Split into four wide bowls.

4. Carnivore Moussaka

It is a high-calorie meal, especially when it comes to high-fat sheep yogurt, aged cheese, and butter. In contrast, please remember that the only thing that contributes carbohydrates to this meal is sheep yogurt. Suppose when it falls to the taste. Just try this recipe because it can satisfy your tastebuds.

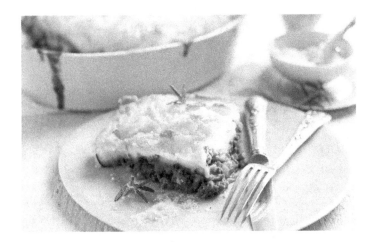

Prep Time: 30 minutes

Cooking Time: 40 minutes

Servings: 4

INGREDIENTS

- 250g (8,8 oz) chopped lamb.

- 250g (8.8 oz) diced beef or veal.

- Eight medium eggs

- 400g (14 oz) Sheep yogurt – strained Greek type (As a substitute use sour cream)

- 500g (1 Lb.) thin veal cutlets

- 50g (1,7 oz) butter or ghee (we always use sheep or goat butter)

- 100g shredded kefalograviera cheese

Spice mixture (amounts to your liking)

- powder rosemary

- dry oregano

- red, white, and black pepper freshly ground.

- dry peppermint

- smoked red paprika powder.

- Ceylon cinnamon

- garlic powder

- sea salt

- ground bay leaves

Instructions

1. Get your chopped meat layer prepared first. In a saucepan or deep-frying pan, dissolve the butter and brown your meat paste in it. Put all the seasoning, except for the oregano, from the list to your taste. In the final moment, you can put oregano so that it does not get sour. Take from heat once the meat sauce is prepared and add one egg. Stir rapidly. Set it down.

2. Roll the veal cutlets with either a sliding pin Grease some butter or ghee to ceramic baking dish or clay.

3. Using a pinch of pepper and sea salt to mix one egg. Dip the egg into each veal slice and put that on the base of the baking dish.

4. Bake at 180oC (350oF) for 10 minutes in the oven.

5. Mix the sheep yogurt or sour cream with six eggs use an electric blender. To your taste, add a pinch of salt.

6. Put the meat sauce over the veal's slices and put the Carnivore moussaka back in the oven. Around ten min, bake. Then coat it with the paste of yogurt or cream and eggs and move it to the oven. Proceed to bake for the next 10 minutes.

7. Then coat it with finely chopped Kefalograviera cheese and layer it uniformly. Please put it back in the oven and cook for ten more minutes. By switching on just the upper heater in the oven, you may use the top process roasting.

8. Represent with a little more finely chopped cheese or a little bit more sour cream. Using fresh parsley or some other texture.

NOTES

You can only use chopped meat sauce for a slightly quicker recipe and cover it with cheese and fluffy topping.

Do not slice till it has cool down at least half the way. It will help you to slice sharp sides with neat pieces.

5. AIP Chicken Bacon Sauté

A delight for the Carnivore's diet: These

AIP chicken bacon sautés indeed a tasty dish that gratifies and best serves you.

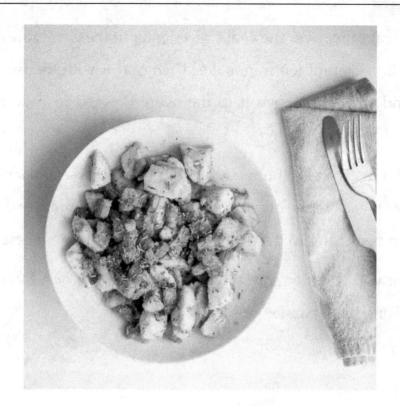

Prep Time: 10 minutes

Cook Time: 20 minutes

Servings: 2

INGREDIENTS

- Four pieces of bacon, diced.

- One tbsp. garlic powder

- One tbsp avocado oil for cooking

- One chicken breast small diced.

- Salt according to taste.

- 2 tbsps. Italian seasoning

INSTRUCTIONS

1. In a frying pan, add the avocado oil and cook the bacon and chicken. Cooked for approximately 10 min.

2. For seasoning, use Italian seasoning, garlic powder and salt according to your taste.

Point to note All nutrition information is calculated and concentrated on quantities per serving.

94. 6. Low Carb Carnitas

Cooked at home carnitas enjoyed with freshly chopped avocados and crunchy onions a quick low carb meal, but it can be a meal memory pretty fast! It is indeed chosen easily to low-carb lifestyle choices, and this carnitas is so delicious that tortillas ought not to be missed in the end.

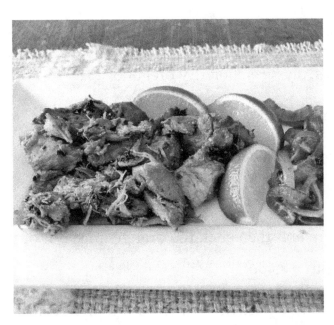

Prep Time: 30 minutes

Cook Time: 2 hrs. 15 minutes.

Servings: 10

Ingredients

- 3 lb. boneless pork shoulder roast cut into 1–2-inch pieces.

- Four sprigs of fresh thyme

- Two cups of water.

- Half cup finely diced onion.

- One teaspoon chipotle spice chooses the spice that suits your taste.

- One orange.

- Prefer one tablespoon lard or oil.

- Two tablespoon lard olive oil if you don't want lard.

- Two bay leaves, one teaspoon dry oregano

- One teaspoon salt.

- Three cloves garlic finely diced.

Instructions

1. Take the orange and then suck the orange juice out of it. In a bowl, bring it together and put it aside.

2. Heat 2 tablespoons of lard above medium-high heat in a heavy bottom pot or large Dutch oven. To line the pot's base, put some sliced meat in one layer, be careful not to create a mess. Cook the first layer of meat till it is browned, flipping both sides brown using tongs. Transfer to a plate if that meat layer is

browned and apply the new layer of meat and cook till browned, then switch to the plate. Rinse until all the meat is browned, then modify.

3. Add the garlic and onion to the Dutch oven pot when the meat is browned, then take away from the pan. Cooked for about 5 minutes or so, frequently mixing, till the onions are crispy and crunchy. Getting back to meat.

4. Utilize the preserved orange zest and juice to the Dutch oven and the next six ingredients (through the Chile pepper). Take it to a boil, lower the heat and cover it. For 2 hours, boil.

5. Take the pot back to a gentle simmer after 2 hours and cook disclosed for 15 to 20 minutes or until most of the liquid has vanished, moving constantly. Take away the bay leaves and thyme sprigs and go to the next stage or store the meat till it is ready. The meat can be stored in the fridge for up to 3 days at this stage.

6. Heat One Tablespoon of lard over the moderate temperature in a big skillet while cooking the carnitas. Remove the meat from the sauce using a slotted spoon and place it over a thin line in the skillet. Cooked for five min or till the meat begins to crust, slightly flipping (you may need to do this in batches).

7. Offer with lime wedges, guacamole (or sliced fresh avocados), refried beans, jalapeno pepper, lime wedges, and caramelized onions.

95. 7. Carnivore's Lasagna

For meat lovers, it is stuffed with Italian sausage, ground beef, meatballs, and pepperoni.

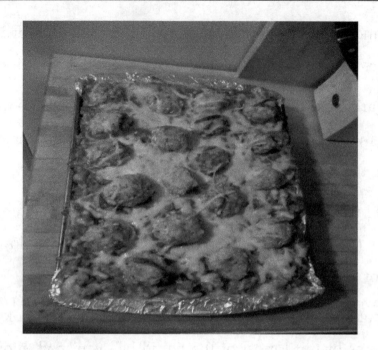

Prep Time: 1 hour 10 minutes.

Cook Time: 1 hour.

Servings: 1 lasagna

INGREDIENTS

- Half onion finely chopped.

- 1 lb. hot Italian sausage sliced.

- Four garlic cloves crumbled.

- 1 1/2 cups parmesan cheese, grated.

- One tsp. Dry oregano, divided.

- 1/2 cup oatmeal

- 3 (15 ounce) cans tomato sauce

- 2 tbsps. Brown sugar

- 18 lasagna noodles

- One tbsp. Fennel seed, divided.

- One tsp. Dried thyme, divided.

- Two lbs. Lean ground beef, divided.

- Two tsps. Salt, divided.

- One tbsp. Olive oil

- One tsp. Black pepper.

- One tsp. Dry basil, divided.

- 2/3 lb. Pepperoni chopped into small pieces.

- Two tbsps. Dry parsley, divided.

- Two eggs.

- 32 ounces ricotta cheese

- Half tsp. ground nutmeg

- 8 -16 ounces mozzarella cheese, grated.

Instructions

1. Heat the oven to 350 degrees.

2. Heat the olive oil in a large pan at moderate temperature. Put garlic, onion, Italian sausage, and half of the ground meat. Cook for approximately 10 minutes.

3. If required, remove the meat mixture. Put 1/2 teaspoon basil, thyme, oregano, fennel seed, salt, black pepper and 1tbsp of brown sugar, one

tablespoon parsley, tomato sauce. Mix, carefully wrap and allow to boil for 1 hour on low flame.

4. Start preparing the ricotta cheese mixture, lasagna noodles and meatballs while the sauce is cooking. Then, in a wide bowl, break one egg. Add the 1/2 cup of Parmesan, oatmeal and the remaining ground meat, basil, fennel, black pepper, thyme, oregano, and salt according to your taste. Merge properly.

5. Shape the meat into balls that have a size of around 1 inch. Please put it on a sprayed pan and bake for 20 minutes, rotating half the way through the cooking time over the meatballs. In the bowl, put the ricotta cheese in it. Add the remaining nutmeg, egg, and the remaining parsley. Merge and set it aside.

6. Then, boil the lasagna noodles for at least 15 minutes in a big pan full of very hot water.

7. The lasagna is placed in a deep 9x3-inch pan till the sauce is cooked. On the base of the pan, pour 2 cups of the sauce. Just lay down six noodles. Layer half of the ricotta on the noodles and top with 1/3 of the parmesan and mozzarella. Place half the pepperoni on top of that.

8. Similarly, make another layer, beginning with 2 cups of sauce. Lay down the remaining portion of the lasagna noodles on top afterward.

9. Blend the rest of the sauce into the cooked meatballs and scatter on top of the lasagna. Cover with a cheese layer.

10. Wrap in foil and bake for 25 minutes at 350F. Let us remove the foil and bake for 25 minutes. Take it out and cool it for 15 minutes before served.

Conclusion

If you've made it on the carnivore diet this far, you finally are noticing some beneficial effects. As a result of your metabolism having shifted completely to ketosis and blood sugar levels remaining consistent, you can feel a lot more physically active with excessive concentration levels. When you undergo the carnivore diet, this is what happens to your body.

While being on the carnivore diet, some individuals even undergo blood sugar drops because carbohydrates' consumption is inaccurate. For patients with Type 2 diabetes, this has to be a preventative measure.

You should also find that one's desires for high carbohydrates will have decreased because you are now better prepared to get all the energy from protein and fat you want.

Rebuild and create every cell in the body; meat has all the nine essential amino acids you consume. And it has some other good things that you will need, too.

Josh Axe, DC, DNM, CNS, and author of Eat Dirt, says that meat is filled with vitamin B12, a nutrient vital for generating long-lasting strength. "Meat also provides your body with a variety of other essential vitamins and minerals many of which are more bioavailable and easier to absorb than the nutrients found in plant sources." There are plant-based foods, of course, as most vegans will say, containing all the essential nutrients (quinoa, for example), and you can combine foods to get everything you need.

Reasonably Set Your Goals

Stick to them and make them accessible. Later or Sooner, you will be confronted with all of the delicious carnivore diet recipes in the world. This one needs a serious effort, like any permissive form of diet. Look ahead, choose the meals for the entire week in advance, and make a grocery list and keep to it as much as practicable to avoid cravings.

Don't start with very wide segments. Although the carnivore diet is in the form of "eat until fulfilled," that does not mean you should strive to explore, especially if weight loss is your target. Go gently and, if necessary, raise the quantities. Using your meal plan as an opportunity to listen more closely to your body's needs, avoiding what it doesn't want.

The Carnivore Diet meal plan will help you meet your goals safely and sustainably if you want to boost your health by avoiding refined foods, achieve your gym goals by underpaying your calorie intake or can't get enough meat.

Wood Pellet Smoker Grill Cookbook

Discover Tens of Succulent Recipes and Learn 9+1 Beginners Tricks to Make Your First Grills with No Pressure

By

Chef Marcello Ruby

Table of Contents

INTRODUCTION   **236**

CHAPTER 1- WOOD PELLET SMOKER GRILLS   **238**

1.1   WHAT IS A PELLET SMOKER GRILL?.. 238
1.2   WORKING OF A PELLET SMOKER GRILL 239
1.3   BASIC COMPONENTS OF A WOOD PELLET SMOKER............................ 240
1.4   USING YOUR WOOD PELLET SMOKER GRILL 244

CHAPTER 2-TRICKS AND TECHNIQUES   **250**

2.1   QUALITY MEAT AND SEASONINGS 250
2.2   USDA MINIMUM INTERNAL TEMPERATURES 251
2.3   GENERAL INFORMATION AND TIPS 254
2.4   SIMPLE TRICKS FOR BEGINNERS 258

CHAPTER 3-APPETIZERS RECIPES   **262**

3.1 ATOMIC BUFFALO TURDS.. 262
3.2 GARLIC PARMESAN WEDGES 263
3.3 BACON-WRAPPED ASPARAGUS... 265
3.4 BOURBON BBQ SMOKED CHICKEN WINGS 265
3.5   BRISKET BAKED BEANS.. 268
3.6   CRABMEAT-STUFFED MUSHROOMS 269
3.7   HICKORY-SMOKED MOINK BALL SKEWERS 271
3.8   SMASHED POTATO CASSEROLE 272
3.9   ROASTED VEGETABLES 274
3.10   APPLEWOOD-SMOKED CHEESE... 275
3.11   BACON CHEDDAR SLIDERS 276
3.12   TERIYAKI STEAK BITES 278

CHAPTER 4-LUNCH RECIPES   **280**

4.1   JAN'S GRILLED QUARTERS... 280
4.2   CAJUN SPATCHCOCK CHICKEN 281
4.3   SMOKED PORK TENDERLOINS 282
4.4   PELLET GRILL SMOKEHOUSE BURGER.. 283
4.5   ROASTED LEG OF LAMB.. 285
4.6   TERIYAKI SMOKED DRUMSTICKS.. 286
4.7   APPLEWOOD WALNUT-CRUSTED RACK OF LAMB.............................. 287
4.8   HOT-SMOKED TERIYAKI TUNA 289

4.9 BAKED FRESH WILD SOCKEYE SALMON 289

4.10 BACON CORDON BLEU 290

4.11 PULLED HICKORY-SMOKED PORK BUTTS 292

4.12 PELLET GRILL PORK LOIN WITH SALSA VERDE 293

CHAPTER 5-DINNER RECIPES   296

5.1 ROASTED TUSCAN THIGHS 296

5.2 SMOKED BONE-IN TURKEY BREAST 297

5.3 CRAB-STUFFED LEMON CORNISH HENS 298

5.4 DOUBLE-SMOKED HAM 299

5.5 EASY NO-FAIL PELLET SMOKER RIBS 300

5.6 TEXAS-STYLE BRISKET FLAT 301

5.7 HICKORY-SMOKED PRIME RIB OF PORK 302

5.8 MEATY CHUCK SHORT RIBS 303

5.9 ROASTED DUCK À I' ORANGE 304

5.10 PETEIZZA MEATLOAF 306

5.11 SHRIMP-STUFFED TILAPIA 308

5.12 EASY SMOKED CHICKEN BREASTS 310

CONCLUSION   312

Introduction

The hottest trend in the BBQ and grilling community have been pellet grills. Since technology has not really improved much in the industry in the last three decades or so, individuals are enthusiastic about the amazing functionality and comfort that pellet grills are bringing to the sector. However, it's crucial to learn how they function in order to fully appreciate what they have to deliver. So, if you're new to grilling or smoking pellets and you're thinking about how pellet grills operate, then you've come to the right place.

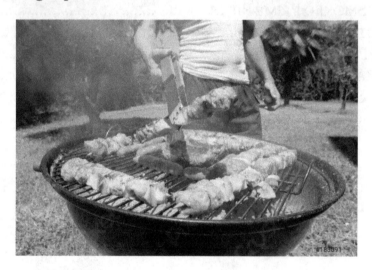

Barbecuing is the oldest form of cooking worldwide. Low-and-slow smoking and cooking over indirect heat is the standard concept of barbecuing. There is little question regarding the findings obtained from barbecuing utilizing haze, indirect fire, sauces, rubs, and natural meat juices. Among grilling and barbecuing, there is a big distinction, but many people are ignorant because they use all words loosely.

Smoker-grills with wood pellets is ideal units for barbecuing.

In this book, you will get to know each and everything you need to learn about the know-how of a Wood Pellet Smoker Grill.

This book provides you with various tips and tricks that you need to know in order to enjoy the process of barbequing and making it a deliciously funny activity.

Also, various basic recipes are provided for you to start with your grilling with ease in the comfort of your home.

Chapter 1- Wood Pellet Smoker Grills

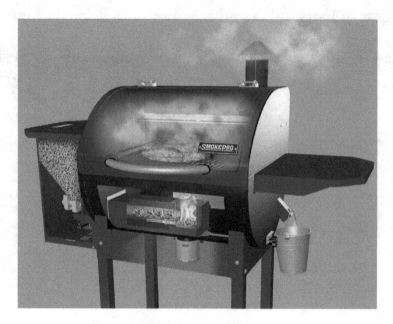

1.1   What is a Pellet Smoker Grill?

A barbecue pit using compressed hardwood sawdust such as apple, plum, hickory, pine, oak, mesquite, and other wood pellets to roast, grill, smoke and bake is the clinical concept of a wood pellet smoker-grill. The smoker-grill wood pellet provides you with taste profiles and moisture that can only be obtained through hardwood cooking. Grill temperatures on certain versions vary from 150 °F to well over 600 °F, depending on the maker and platform.

Wood pellet smoker-grills are succulent, cosy and clean, unparalleled by gas grills and charcoal. The smoke composition is milder than you may be accustomed to from other cigarettes. They produce the flexibility and advantages of a convection oven due to their architecture. Smoker-grills with wood pellets is safe and easy to work.

In short outdoor cookers that incorporate components from smokers, kitchen ovens, charcoal smokers, and gas grills are pellet grills. They use 100% of natural hardwood pellets, the fuel supply that enables direct or indirect heat to be generated by Pellet Grills.

Fueled by wood pellets, utilizing an electronic control panel, they will smoke and grill and bake to automatically feed fuel pellets to the flames, regulate the ventilation of the grill, and maintain constant cooking temperatures.

1.2   Working of a Pellet Smoker Grill

Wood pellets are placed into a hopper-called storage container. An auger that is operated by electricity then feeds the pellets into a cooking chamber. The wood pellets ignite by combustion, warming the cooking chamber. After that, the air is pulled in by intake fans. Across the boiling area, flame and smoke are then emitted.

Rather like an oven, pellet grills provide you digitally or with a knob with reliable temperature regulation, typically varying from 180 ° F to 500 ° F. So, "low and slow" or searing hot both can be cooked by you.

In order to check the core temperature of the beef, most pellet grills do have a meat probe that can link with the control board. There is a proprietary Sear Zone plate for grills that requires implicit or explicit heat and eight separate cooking methods.

1.3   Basic Components of a Wood Pellet Smoker

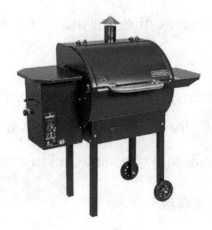

The following provided are the basic components of a wood pellet smoker grill: -

1.   Hopper

This is where they store the wood pellets. Be sure you hold a good quantity of pellets based on the cook's range, the cook's temperature, and the capability of the hopper.

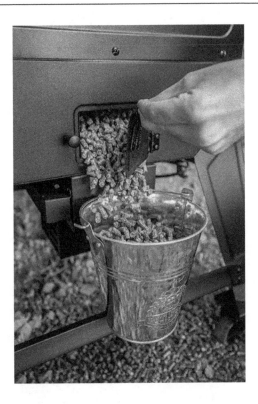

2.   Firepot

This is where the fire and burn the wood pellets that ignite the barbecue. For the pellet shaft, which holds the auger, the wide hole in the firepot is; the bottom center gap below it is for the igniter tube, and the other holes are for the ventilation of the fan. After a few cooks, it is a good idea to empty or vacuum out the ashes in order to enable the igniter to function more effectively.

3.   Auger

The pellets are then loaded via the auger, the feed system that provides the fire pot with the pellets.

4.   Fan

As it ensures a constant and/or steady airflow, the fan is very critical, maintaining the pellets trying to burn in the firepot and culminating in cooking convection.

5.   Igniter Rod

The wood pellets are ignited in the firepot by this rod. The ignitor rod and the pellet feed tube that is required by the auger to supply pellets to the firepot can be seen with the firepot away.

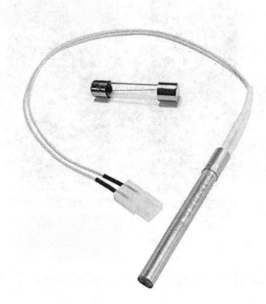

6.   Hear Deflector

A specially crafted plate covering the firepot is the heat deflector. The goal is to absorb the heat and distribute it uniformly under the grease/drip plate, converting the wood pellet smoker-grill into a wood-fired convection oven effectively.

7.   Resistive Temperature Detector (RTD) / Thermocouple

The thermal sensor that supplies the input loop to the controller is the RTD or thermocouple. For better heat readings, deep clean the thermocouple regularly.

8.   Flame Zone Pan

For clear, high-temperature grilling, it is used in tandem with searing grates and attachments for the griddle.

9.   Drip Pan

In indirect frying, smoking, baking and roasting, the oiled pan is used. It routes the grease generated to the grease bucket during cooking. It is recommended to scrape off an appropriate caked-on residue from cooks. Also, substitute the foil per few cooks if utilizing foil.

10.   Grease Bucket

Runoff fat and oil from cooking activities are extracted from the grease bucket. Accumulation of grease relies on how often you want to cut from beef and poultry fat caps and extra fat. Lining the foil grease bowl tends you clear up.

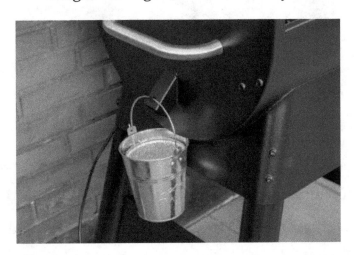

11.   Controller

To preserve the set-point temperature, the controller, which normally comes in several types, regulates the air and pellet movement.

1.4   Using your Wood Pellet Smoker Grill

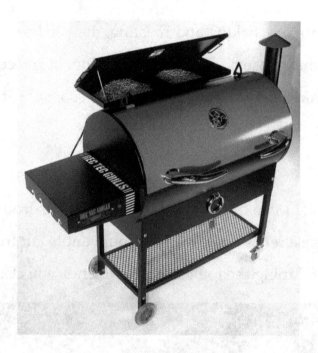

1.   Assembly

If a nearby distributor assembles your product for you or you order your unit from a big box retailer, you will need to install your wood pellet smoker-grill. Whether you order the product directly from the vendor or via an online distributor, the unit would also be shipped on a pallet by a ground carrier. But don't dread; assembly isn't as rough as it seems or as complicated as you would imagine.

Only set out all of the bits, and yes, before you begin assembly, make sure you read the directions. Tech help and assistance are just a phone call away, and several suppliers have excellent customer care.

You'll find the design and directions will help you to create your smoker-grill wood pellet easily in an hour or less. In most units, the foundation and legs are often mounted. You will have your device full of wood pellets and ready for the initial burn-in in no time. Be sure you have someone to support you if and where the directions ask for two persons. By choosing to do things yourself, do not harm yourself.

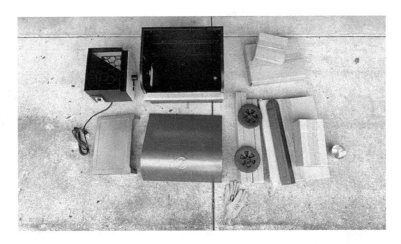

2. Ignition

Wood pellet smoker-grills require standard household 120 VAC or 12 VDC outlets. For powering the ignition and service, wood pellet smoker-grills require regular household 120 VAC or 12 VDC outlets. For, e.g., certain devices, such as the Davy Crockett tailgate device from Green Mountain Grills, are built to use 12 VDC from a car battery or a deep-cycle battery. They also have a 120 VAC AC/DC converter for usage. The power requirements are actually very limited for wood pellet smoker-grills and are used for four items: fan, auger, controller and igniter rod.

Smoker-grills with wood pellets are very safe and easy to work. Inside the fire pot, the fire/flames are limited and completely protected by the oil pan, which gives indirect cooking and avoids flare-ups. Typically, based on the maker, one of two factors can arise when you turn on your device. Your pit either goes through a particular power-up series, or a typical scenario follows it.

The controller is flipped on, the igniter rod is triggered (it will glow red hot), the auger feeds a certain volume of pellets into the firepot, and the fan feeds air into the firepot through numerous tiny holes to start and sustain the fire. The igniter rod is either switched off after a fixed period (4 minutes or longer) or when the pit exceeds a set temperature, depending on your controller. To stop flame-outs, PID controllers can switch the igniter rod back on when the temperature falls below a fixed temperature.

3.   Initial Burn-In

To burn out all oils and chemicals used in the processing phase, the burn-in technique is used.

With hardwood barbecue-grade wood pellets, fill the hopper. Because the transmission of the first pellets to the firepot can take ten or more minutes for the auger, put half a handful of pellets in the firepot. Attach the device into a 120 VAC electrical socket with grounding. Just turn on your grill. Place temperature between 350 ° F and 450 ° F if you have a digital controller, and allow the grill to operate at temperature for 30 to 60 minutes (check your owner's manual for precise temperature settings and time). Convert the temperature setting to strong if your grill has an LMH controller.

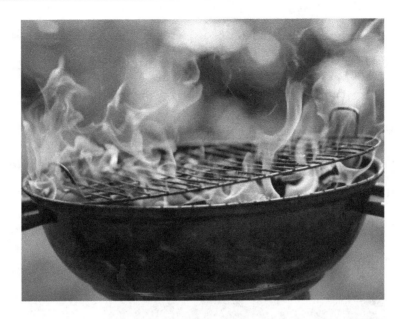

4.   Testing for Hot Spots on Your Wood Pellet Smoker-Grill

Not all wood pellet smoker-grills are identical, but I promise that you will be able to smoke and prepare some of the best food your family and friends will ever experience by knowing about your barbecue! To have a working knowledge of the barbecue, it just takes a few cooks to train.

You'll want to monitor the temperature of the grill surface for uniform heat and hotspots. The biscuit test is one simple way to do this.

In the corners, front, back, and middle of the barbecue pick up a box of refrigerator biscuits and position them. As per the instructions on the box, cook the biscuits. You can discover where the hotter and colder places are in your device with this exercise.

Place your food and prepare it according to the data you've gained.

The use of a remote temperature probe to measure the temperatures at the same positions as the biscuit test is needed for a more technical process. At each biscuit spot, put a remote temperature probe, check the temperature, contrast it to the fixed point on your controller and, if any, record the temperature variations. No matter how nice your grill controller is, regardless of the position of the RTD/thermocouple, you'll notice discrepancies. To attain the temperatures you like, just change your grill's fixed temperatures accordingly.

5. Cleaning Your Wood Pellet Smoker-Grill

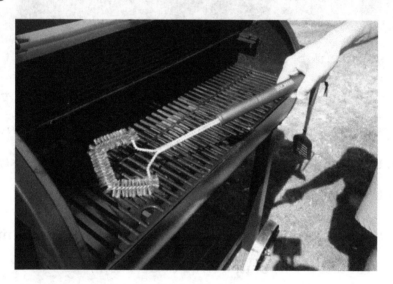

It is highly recommended that you keep your smoker-grill with wood pellets as clean as possible. It only takes a couple of minutes to keep the pit clean before you cook. Cleanliness ensures that your cooks are always penetrated with fresh and clean smoke. For the best results, after every hard cook or after every two to four short cooks, replace the foil on the grease drop pan. If you choose not to use foil, then make sure that the caked residue is often scraped off from your drip pan. There is nothing other than the gases burning off at elevated temperatures from rancid old grease. Using a barbecue wire brush to scrub and hold them clean after each cooker, when the grill grates are still hot. Wipe down both sides of the grates using paper towels. When handling the grates and cleaning your pit, I strongly suggest you wear disposable rubber gloves.

Once your pit fully cools down, remove the drip pan and regularly remove any ash from the firepot and the body of the pit using a shop vacuum cleaner. Although smoker-grills with wood pellets are incredibly effective, you will still accumulate some ash.

Large quantities of ash in the firepot will decrease the unit's efficiency and might not cause the igniter rod to ignite pellets properly at star-tup. During a roast, an ash accumulation in the body of the pit has a chance to be blown around and collected on the beef.

Chapter 2-Tricks and Techniques

2.1   Quality Meat and Seasonings

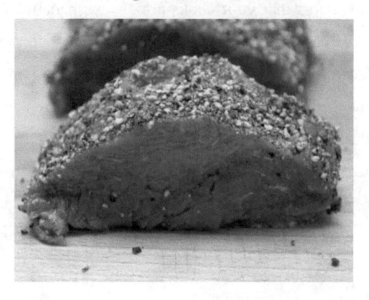

For excellent and personalized cuts of meats, sausages and poultry, and as well as wonderful rubs, seasonings, and barbecue sauces, don't forget your friendly neighbourhood butcher shop.

Low-and-slow cooking, grilling, smoking, frying, roasting, etc., are always worth the seasoning.

It is strongly suggested that you go out and visit the nearest butcher shops and meat markets to see if you can even locate the jewel in the rough that will create an excellent crowd of your next chef.

FTC-In order to redistribute the juices into the product, this significant acronym stands for "Foil-Towel-Cooler" and is a popular process used for retaining and/or resting cooked meats, such as pork butts, turkey and brisket. It provides a final product that is juicy and tender. For example, to accomplish these effects, pit masters, professionals, caterers, and restaurants utilize industrial units such as a Cambro. The FTC is lovingly referred to as the Cambro of the unfortunate guy.

To hold the juices contained, double-wrap the cooked meat in heavy-duty aluminium foil. Before you put it in a cooler, cover the foiled meat in a wide towel. Minimize air room if needed by covering the majority of the cooler with towels to help prevent the heat from dissipating. Depending on the meat and/or the period available before serving, FTC pork butts and briskets are processed in a locked cooler for a minimum of 2 hours and up to 4 to 6 hours. When processing meat, take care, since it may always be too hot to handle even after resting for hours.

2.2   USDA Minimum Internal Temperatures

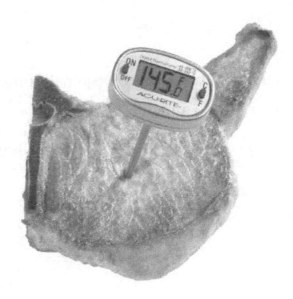

As determined with an automated food thermometer, cook all food at these required internal temperatures before extracting it from the heat source. For purposes of personal choice, you can choose to cook at higher temperatures.

1.   Indirect and Direct Grill Setup

Both smoker-grills with wood pellets are built mainly for indirect cooking. To cook more slowly and uniformly, indirect cooking utilizes deflected fire. The heat deflector is a stainless-steel plate that sits above the fire pot, as described before. It collects the heat from the fire and radiates it out like a convection oven does, ensuring that the heat is spread around it, giving a cook that is more uniform. Direct cooking uses direct, high heat to cook, much as the name suggests. It's a quicker time to cook, which doesn't make for many infusions of smoke, but it does give you the iconic grill marks. More producers are now starting to provide the versatility of a direct cooking setup, and a limited number have a built-in hybrid design that both offers indirect and direct cooking power without needing to alter any configuration.

- **Indirect Setup**

You'll be using an indirect rig for several wood pellet smoker-grill recipes. Per your manufacturer's user manual, mount your grease pan. In order for the grease fat to fall out, the Grease pan is built to slant in the path of the grease bucket. Otherwise, at higher temperatures, the grease would collect on the pan, which might become a flare-up safety problem.

- **Direct Setup**

You will need to swap your indirect pan with a direct pan because your machine has built-in direct cooking capabilities. To customize it for direct cooking, you can need to detach one or more cover plates in certain units or slip the top part of a combination pan. To close or expose the gaps, you slip the cover in one direction or the other. Shuttered holes are for indirect cooking, whereas direct cooking is for open holes. Searing gratings are not obligatory. They can have greater results when grilling and cooking directly since they are built to sear and sizzle foods easier by focusing the fire.

2.   Ingredients

Feel free to replace, delete, and incorporate some ingredients dependent on your tastes, taste buds, and ingredients on hand, depending on how relaxed you are in the kitchen or with the grill. Strict adherence to the list of ingredients can deliver impressive results, but do not be afraid to tweak it here and there.

3.   Prepping for the Grill

Before taking the food to the barbecue, the prep portion is all the preparation you do. Planning ahead is the number one goal in the prep period. Offer yourself plenty of time, read the recipe, and examine every move or process in which you can have concerns. To allow the seasonings, rubs, marinades and brines to do their magic, recipes can call for refrigeration overnight or for hours after making preparations. Before beginning your preparation, gather all required ingredients and cooking equipment. Before starting, make sure the proteins are safely thawed in the refrigerator if you do not use fresh beef, poultry, or seafood. Be vigilant to have good sanitary facilities, above all.

There may be occasions when the processes of planning and guidance can occur concurrently. You may opt to preheat before finishing the cooking, based on the length of time your wood pellet smoker-grill needs to preheat, much as in a conventional indoor oven.

4. On the Wood Pellet Smoker Grill

Unless otherwise stated, it is strongly recommended to start with a complete pellet hopper and a clean wood pellet smoker-grill configured for indirect fire. If required, prior to putting the meat on the plate, insert the grill meat probe(s) or remote meat probe(s) into the thickest part of the protein. Bear in mind that each smoker grill for wood pellets is different, and so the time to create various recipes may vary accordingly. Depend on internal temperatures at all times. Just to find out that it's undercooked, you won't believe how scrumptious a piece of meat might look.

You can soon discover when you grow confident with your wood pellet smoker-grill that cooking directions can be adjustable as long as the correct internal temperature is met by your finished product.

2.3 General Information and Tips

1. Preheating

According to factory start-up procedures, times for heating up your wood pellet smoker-grill can differ. The trick is to run a few experiments to grasp your barbecue.

2. Thawing Food

Always thaw food in the refrigerator to be healthy to avoid illness; immerse it in freezing water, adjust the water every 30 minutes and ensure that the food remains submerged; or use the freezer to defrost the food. On the countertop, do not thaw the frozen food.

3. Internal Temperature

Often use a wireless instant-read thermometer such as a Thermapen or an analogous device to cook at internal temperatures. Before putting the protein on the grill, probe thermometers should be inserted and put in the thickest section of the beef, not reaching the bone.

4. Tenting

Until slicing or eating, many recipes ask for resting the meat under a foil tent. Tenting is a simple process.

In the middle, fold sheets of aluminium foil, fan it opens into a tent form and position it loosely over the food. Instead of placing them on the serving tray, tenting tends to preserve heat as the food redistributes the natural juices. By tenting, crispy skin texture on poultry and crisp on meats may be affected.

5. The Stall

A natural part of the cooking process is the stall, also known as the plateau or zone. Large cuts of meat reach a point when cooked at low temperatures, where the core temperature stops rising for a period of time. After the collagen melts, most cuts of meat tenderize, and the fibres begin to separate. The stall will experience every big chunk of meat, such as a pork butt (shoulder) or beef brisket. It can last minutes or as long as three hours and normally occurs from 155 ° F to 170 ° F at internal meat temperatures. It's not a question of whether, but when, the stall is going to happen. In your wood pellet smoker-grill, you may be tempted to turn the heat up, but practice patience; just ride it out so as not to affect the meat being cooked.

6. The Texas Crutch

A technique is commonly known as the "Texas crutch" will decrease your cooking time and bypass the stall for those who cannot wait out the stall. The most preferred version of the Texas crutch is to consider removing the meat from the stall before it reaches its full size. When the internal temperature reaches 160 °F, remove the meat, then double wrap it in heavy-duty aluminium foil, ensuring that any meat probes are inserted into the meat. Wrap the foil around the probe until it attains your desired internal temperature, and return the meat to the grill.

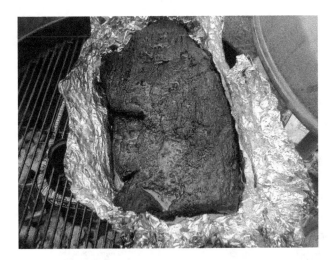

7. Carving Meat

Always carve meat across the grain, not with it, to get the most tender outcomes. Searching for the simultaneous lines running down the meat identifies the direction that the grain is running. Slice the muscle fibre lines perpendicular to them.

8. Protect your Skin

While handling raw meat and spicy peppers like jalapeños, wear food-grade latex-free nitric gloves.

9. Keep your Prep Surface Clean

It is highly recommended that plastic food wrap and/or heavy-duty aluminium foil line your prep area. When dealing with raw meat, this simplifies clean-up and is also more hygienic.

10. Curing Salt

Curing salt contains salt and nitrite, which is used in some low-and-slow recipes and should not be used to season food at the table or during the cooking process. Significant quantities can be lethal, but when curing meat, it is harmless in small quantities.

11.   Smoke Issues

The higher the temperature, the lower smoke is produced by a wood pellet smoker-grill. No noticeable smoke above 300°F will be produced by most units. Therefore, when a recipe initially calls for extremely high temperatures, use any pellets of your choice, as the pellets will not influence the flavour.

2.4   Simple tricks for beginners

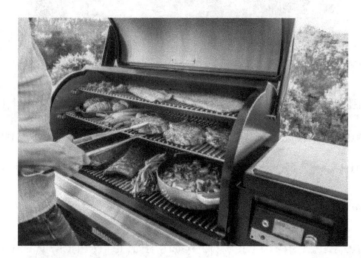

1.   Allow yourself some time to get acquainted with your new grill/smoker

Allow yourself time to familiarize yourself with your new grill/smoker. We know you're going to be anxious to give it a try, but don't be overly ambitious. Start with chicken, salmon steaks or fillets, pork loin tenderloin, Cornish hens, blade steaks, or other fairly affordable cuts that can be completed in 2 hours or less, instead of a whole brisket that might take 15 hours or more, or a budget-busting prime rib roast.

2.   Don't let your meat come to room temperature before cooking

Whichever meat you select, put it straight from the refrigerator on the preheated grill/smoker. Do not allow it to reach room temperature before cooking, as many recipes suggest.

3.   Take advantage of your pellet grill's searing capabilities

Many pellet grills feature searing capabilities, which means that temperatures above 500 °C can be reached. Again, for information on your particular model, check your owner's manual.

4.   Use the reverse sear method

Don't think about smoking the meat at a lower temperature and then finishing it at a high temperature. This two-step approach is particularly useful for smoking crisp (not rubbery) skin chicken, or the "reverse sear technique" often used for thicker steaks or prime ribs.

5.   Use your pellet grill just like an oven

Just like an oven, your smoker/pellet grill can be used, capable of baking, roasting, braising, etc. But the inclusion of wood smoke gives much more fascinating flavours to food.

6.   Experiment with pellet flavours

Experiment with the flavours of pellets. Certain pellet labels are somewhat subtle.

7.   Position your grill at least 6 feet away from your home

At least six feet from any buildings, overhangs, bushes, etc., place your barbecue.

8.   Always store pellets in a dry place

Pellets can always be kept in a dry spot. Otherwise, it'll transform to sawdust, and if it's an augur, to anything like a stone!

9. Use the upper rack of your grill for cooking something that's prone to drying out

Convection and radiant heat are also generated by your pellet grill. Place them on the upper rack to shield them from the heat radiating from the bottom while you are frying anything that is vulnerable to drying out, such as thin fish fillets or chicken breasts. You can balance a wire rack on fire bricks or buy after-market racks if your machine doesn't come with an upper rack. To produce moisture, you may also place a pan of water or other liquid on the grill grate.

10. Season your new pellet grill

Season your new pellet grill according to directions from the manufacturer. This burns off the production process of any residual oils.

11. Identify any hot spots — most grills have them

As directed by the owner's manual, preheat your grill to medium-high, then lay slices of cheap white bread shoulder to shoulder across the grater. Watch carefully, then after a couple of minutes, flip. Take a photo of the findings. The darkest bread will show where the temperature could be warmer

12. Invest in a good meat thermometer

At grill level, a laser-type thermometer will give you a more precise temperature reading than an integrated dome thermometer. Determine your grill model's temperature range from lowest to highest.

13. Use lower temperatures to generate more smoke

At lower temperatures, especially in the "low and slow" range between 225 and 275, you will generate more smoke.

14.   Never allow the pellets in the pellet hopper to run out

Never allow it to run out of the pellets in the pellet hopper. If this occurs, before relighting the barbecue, check the owner's manual. To reassure yourself to top off the pellets, set a timer if you have to.

15.   Invest in a smoking tube to supplement the smoke generated by your grill

If you want to complement your pellet grill with the smoke produced, or even cold smoke, engage in a smoking tube.

16.   Clean your grill frequently

To prevent the build-up of ash or oil, clean your grill regularly. Much like a sharp-bladed spatula or putty knife, a shop-type vacuum is a must. Don't neglect to sweep the exhaust or chimney.

17.   Use heavy-duty foil for easier clean-up

To protect the oil tray and to line the grease bucket, use high-duty foil. (Also, hollow containers may be used as bucket liners, such as coffee or tomato cans.)

18.   Remove the grease bucket after each cook

Take the grease bucket off the side of the grill after each cooker and hide it in a secure position to keep it out of the hands of pets, coyotes or other hungry creatures.

19.   Smoke vegetables and side dishes on your new grill

Using the new grill to smoke or roast vegetables or side dishes.

Chapter 3-Appetizers Recipes

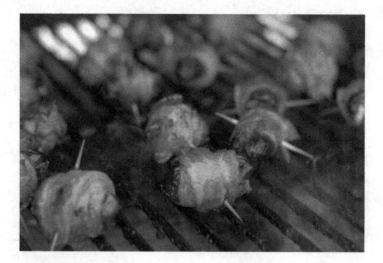

3.1 Atomic Buffalo Turds

Ready in about 2 hours and 50 minutes | Servings-6 to 10 | Difficulty-Hard

Ingredients

- 3⁄4 cup of shredded Monterey Jack and cheddar cheese blend

- Half teaspoon of red pepper flakes

- Eight ounces of regular cream cheese

- Ten medium jalapeño peppers

- One teaspoon of garlic powder

- Ten thinly sliced bacon strips, cut in half

- One teaspoon of smoked paprika

- Twenty Little Smokies sausages

- Half teaspoon of cayenne pepper

Instructions

1.   Firstly, if you use your food service gloves, we need to ready the grill for that. Clean the jalapeño peppers and slice them lengthwise. Carefully extract the seeds and veins using a spoon or paring knife, and dispose of them. On a vegetable grilling tray, put the jalapeños and set them aside.

2.   Mix the cream cheese, shredded cheese, paprika, cayenne pepper, garlic powder, and red pepper flakes in a small cup, if using, until they are thoroughly absorbed.

3.   With the cream cheese mixture, cover the hollowed jalapeño pepper pieces.

4.   On top of each half of the packed jalapeño pepper, put a Little Smokies sausage.

5.   Wrap each half of the jalapeño pepper with half a slice of thin bacon.

6.   To secure the bacon to the sausage, use a toothpick, making sure not to pierce the pepper. On a grilling tray or skillet, position the ABTs.

7.   For indirect cooking, set up your wood pellet smoker-grill and preheat it to 250°F using hickory pellets or a mix.

8.   Smoke the jalapeño peppers for one and a half to 2 hours at 250 ° F before the bacon is fried and crunchy.

9.   Remove the ABTs from the grill and leave to rest before serving for 5 minutes.

3.2 Garlic Parmesan Wedges

Ready in about 45 minutes | Servings-3 | Difficulty-Moderate

Ingredients

- A quarter cup of extra-virgin olive oil

- 3⁄4 teaspoon of black pepper

- 3⁄4 cup of grated Parmesan cheese

- Three tablespoons of chopped fresh cilantro

- Three large russet potatoes

- One and a half teaspoons of salt

- Two teaspoons of garlic powder

- Half cup of blue cheese or ranch dressing per serving, for dipping (optional)

Instructions

1.   Using a vegetable brush to gently clean the potatoes with cold water and allow the potatoes to dry.

2.   Lengthwise, cut the potatoes in half and then split both halves into thirds.

3.   To clean away all the humidity that is emitted as you cut the potatoes, use a paper towel. Moisture prevents the wedges from being crispy.

4.   In a wide cup, put the potato wedges, pepper, salt, olive oil, and garlic powder and toss gently with your hands to ensure that the oil and spices are equally spread.

5.   Arrange the wedges on a non-stick grilling tray/pan/basket on a single sheet.

6.   For indirect cooking, set up your wood pellet smoker-grill and preheat it to 425 ° F using any form of wood pellet.

7.   Place your preheated smoker-grill on the grilling tray and roast the potato wedges for Fifteen minutes before turning. Roast the potato wedges until the potatoes are fork-tender on the inside and crunchy golden brown on the outside, for an extra 15 to 20 minutes.

8.   Sprinkle with Parmesan cheese on the potato wedges and garnish with, if needed, cilantro or parsley. If needed, serve with ranch dressing blue cheese for dipping.

3.3 Bacon-Wrapped Asparagus

Ready in about 45 minutes | Servings-4 to 6 | Difficulty-Hard

Ingredients

- Extra-virgin olive oil
- One pound of thick fresh asparagus
- Five slices of thinly sliced bacon
- One teaspoon of Pete's Western Rub
- Salt and pepper as per taste

Instructions

1.   Snap and trim the woody ends of the asparagus so that they are both around the same weight.

2.   Divide the asparagus into three-spear packets and spray it with olive oil. With one slice of bacon, seal each package and then sprinkle with the seasoning or salt and pepper to taste.

3.   Configure your indirect cooking wood pellet smoker-grill, putting Teflon-coated fiberglass mats on top of the grates. Using some kind of pellets, preheat to 400°F. It is possible to preheat the grill when heating the asparagus.

4.   For 25 to 30 minutes, grill the bacon-wrapped asparagus until the asparagus is soft and the bacon is fried and crispy.

3.4 Bourbon BBQ Smoked Chicken Wings

Ready in about 2 hours and 50 minutes | Servings-6 | Difficulty-Hard

Ingredients

Wings

- Sweet and smoky chicken rub or your favorite store-bought rub

- Four pounds of chicken wings

- Two tablespoons of vegetable oil

Bourbon BBQ Sauce

- Five finely minced cloves of garlic

- Half finely minced medium sweet yellow onion

- Half cup of bourbon

- A quarter cup of tomato paste

- Two cups of ketchup

- Half cup of packed light brown sugar

- 1/3 cup apple cider vinegar

- A quarter cup of Worcestershire sauce

- Two tablespoons of liquid smoke

- Half tablespoon of kosher salt

- Half teaspoon of black pepper

- A quarter teaspoon of cayenne pepper

- A few dashes of hot sauce (optional)

Instructions

For sauce

1.   Over medium heat, add a drizzle of olive oil to a saucepan. Add the garlic and onion and cook for about 5 minutes. Add the bourbon and continue cooking for approximately 3 minutes.

2. To break it up, add tomato paste and whisk. Add all the remaining components of the sauce and whisk to combine. Increase the heat and bring it to a boil. Simmer for about 15-20 minutes and reduce the heat to medium-low or low.

3. When you like a smooth, glossy sauce, pour sauce through a fine-mesh sieve to strain out pieces of onion and garlic. Set aside to cool. Store the leftover BBQ sauce for 2-3 weeks in the refrigerator in an airtight container.

For wings

1. Pat dry chicken wings with a clean paper towel. In a large mixing bowl, add the wings and toss with the vegetable oil. Ensure that each wing is coated; add rub and massage into the wings.

2. Add pellets of hickory wood to the hopper. Turn on the smoker, open the lid and set the setting for the smoke. Smoke-free heat, lid open, 5-10 minutes, until very smoky. Set the smoker to 250 F degrees by adding chicken wings to the oiled grill grates. Close the smoker's lid and smoke for 2 hours and 30 minutes, or until the internal temperature of the chicken wings reaches 165 degrees F. To ensure precise cooking temperatures, use an instant reading meat thermometer.

3. With bourbon BBQ sauce, change the smoker setting to high and braise chicken wings on both sides. Cook the wings on the other side for 5 minutes, then flip them over and cook for 3-5 minutes.

4. To remove chicken wings from a foil or parchment coated plate or baking sheet, select Shut down on smoker. Allow 5-10 minutes to rest. Turn it off and unplug the smoker.

5. Eat the wings as they are, or brush them with extra BBQ sauce. Dip in the blue cheese or ranch dressing for a traditional experience and serve with celery and carrots.

3.5   Brisket Baked Beans

Ready in about 2 hours and 30 minutes | Servings-10 to 12 | Difficulty-Hard

Ingredients

- Two tablespoons of extra-virgin olive oil

- One large diced yellow onion,

- One medium diced green bell pepper

- One medium diced red bell pepper

- Two to six diced jalapeño peppers

- Three cups of chopped Texas-Style Brisket Flat

- One (28-ounce) can of baked beans, like Bush's Country Style Baked Beans

- One (28-ounce) can of pork and beans

- One (14-ounce) can of rinsed and drained red kidney beans

- One cup of barbecue sauce

- Half cup of packed brown sugar

- Three chopped garlic cloves

- Two teaspoons of ground mustard

- Half teaspoon of kosher salt

- Half teaspoon of black pepper

Instructions

1.   Heat the olive oil in a skillet over medium heat, and then add the diced onion, peppers and jalapeños. Cook for about 8 to 10 minutes, occasionally stirring, until the onions are translucent.

2.   Combine the chopped brisket, pork, baked beans and beans, cooked onion, kidney beans and peppers, barbecue sauce, brown sugar, ground mustard, garlic, black pepper and salt in a 4-quart casserole dish.

3.   Use the pellets of choice to install your wood pellet smoker-grill for indirect cooking and preheat it to 325 ° F. Cook the uncovered brisket of baked beans for one and a half to 2 hours until the beans are dense and bubbly. Allow 15 minutes to rest before serving.

3.6   Crabmeat-Stuffed Mushrooms

Ready in about 50 minutes | Servings-4 to 6 | Difficulty-Moderate

Ingredients

- Extra-virgin olive oil
- Six medium portobello mushrooms
- 1/3 cup of grated Parmesan cheese

For the crabmeat stuffing

- Two tablespoons of extra-virgin olive oil
- Eight ounces of fresh crabmeat, or canned or imitation crab meat
- 1/3 cup of chopped celery
- 1/3 cup of chopped red bell pepper
- Half cup of chopped green onion
- Half cup of Italian bread crumbs
- Half cup of mayonnaise8 ounces cream cheese, at room temperature
- Half teaspoon of minced garlic
- One tablespoon of dried parsley

- Half cup of grated Parmesan cheese
- A quarter teaspoon of Old Bay seasoning
- A quarter teaspoon of kosher salt
- A quarter teaspoon of black pepper

Instructions

1. Using a damp paper towel, clean the mushroom caps. Cut and set aside the stems.

2. With a spoon, extract the brown gills from the undersides of the mushroom caps and dispose of them.

3. Get the crabmeat stuffing ready. Drain, rinse and remove any shell bits when using canned crabmeat.

4. Heat olive oil over medium-high heat in a skillet. Add the celery, green onion and bell pepper, and sauté for 5 minutes. Set to cool aside.

5. In a large bowl, mix the cooled sautéed vegetables gently with the rest of the ingredients.

6. Cover the crabmeat stuffing and refrigerate it until ready to use.

7. Fill the crab mixture with each mushroom cap, creating a mound in the center.

8. Sprinkle with extra-virgin olive oil and sprinkle the Parmesan cheese with each stuffed mushroom cap. In a 10 x, 15-inch baking dish, put the stuffed mushrooms.

9. Install your wood pellet smoker-grill for indirect heat and use any pellets to preheat to 375 ° F.

10. Bake for 30 to 45 minutes until the stuffing is hot and the mushrooms are beginning to release their juices (165 °F measured with an instant-read digital thermometer).

3.7   Hickory-Smoked Moink Ball Skewers

Ready in about 1 hour and 50 minutes | Servings-6 to 9 | Difficulty-Hard

Ingredients

- Half pound ground pork sausage
- Half pound ground beef
- One large egg
- Half cup of Italian bread crumbs
- Half cup of minced red onions
- Half cup of grated Parmesan cheese
- A quarter cup of finely chopped parsley
- A quarter cup of whole milk
- Two minced garlic cloves
- One teaspoon of oregano
- Half teaspoon of kosher salt
- Half teaspoon of black pepper
- Half pound thinly sliced bacon, cut in half
- A quarter cup of barbecue sauce

Instructions

1.   Combine the ground pork sausage, ground beef, egg, onion, parmesan cheese, bread crumbs, parsley, milk, salt, garlic, oregano, and pepper in a large bowl. Don't overwork the flesh.

2.   Form one and a half-ounce meatball, roughly 1 inch in diameter, and place them on a fiberglass mat coated with Teflon.

3.   Wrap half a slice of thin bacon with each meatball. On six skewers, spear the moink balls (3 balls per skewer)

4.   For indirect cooking, configure your wood pellet smoker-grill.

5.   Using hickory pellets, preheat your wood pellet smoker-grill to 225°F.

6.   For 30 minutes, smoke the Moink Ball Skewers.

7.   Raise the pit temperature to 350 ° F until the internal temperature of the meatballs reaches 175 ° F, and the bacon is crunchy (approximately 40 to 45 minutes).

8.   During the last 5 minutes, brush the moink balls with your favourite barbecuing sauce.

3.8   Smashed Potato Casserole

Ready in about 1 hour and 55 minutes | Servings-8 | Difficulty-Hard

Ingredients

- A quarter cup of (Half stick) salted butter
- Ten bacon slices
- One small thinly sliced red onion
- One small thinly green sliced bell pepper
- One small thinly sliced red bell pepper
- One small thinly sliced yellow bell pepper
- Three cups of mashed potatoes
- 3/4 cup of sour cream
- One and a half teaspoons of Texas Barbecue Rub
- Four cups of frozen hash brown potatoes
- Three cups of shredded sharp cheddar cheese

Instructions

1.   Over medium heat, cook the bacon in a large skillet until crisp, about 5 minutes on each side. Set aside the bacon.

2.   To a glass container, transfer the rendered bacon grease.

3.   Warm the butter or bacon grease in the same large skillet, over medium heat, and sauté the red onion and bell peppers until al dente. Just set aside.

4.   Spray non-stick cooking spray on a 9 to 11-inch casserole dish and spread the mashed potatoes on the bottom of the dish.

5.   Layer the sour cream and season with Texas Barbecue Rub over the mashed potatoes.

6.   On top of the potatoes, layer the sautéed vegetables and keep the butter or bacon grease in the pan.

7.   Sprinkle with half a cup of sharp cheddar cheese, followed by brown potatoes with frozen hash.

8.   Spoon over the hash browns with the residual butter or bacon fat from the sautéed vegetables and top with crumbled bacon.

9.   Top with one and a half of the remaining cups of sharp cheddar cheese and cover with a lid or aluminium foil over the casserole dish.

10.   Use the pellets of choice to customize your wood pellet smoker-grill for indirect cooking and preheat it to 350 ° F.

11.   For 45 to 60 minutes, bake the mashed potato casserole until the cheese is bubbling.

12.   Before serving, let it rest for 10 minutes.

3.9   Roasted Vegetables

Ready in about 1 hour | Servings-4 | Difficulty-Moderate

Ingredients

- One cup of small halved mushrooms
- One medium sliced and halved yellow squash
- One small chopped red onion
- Six medium stemmed asparagus spears
- A quarter cup of roasted garlic–flavoured extra-virgin olive oil
- Three minced garlic cloves
- One teaspoon of dried oregano
- Half teaspoon of black pepper
- One cup of cauliflower florets
- One medium sliced and halved zucchini
- One medium chopped red bell pepper
- Six ounces of small baby carrots
- One cup of cherry or grape tomatoes
- Two tablespoons of balsamic vinegar
- One teaspoon of dried thyme
- One teaspoon of garlic salt

Instructions

1.   Place in a large bowl the florets of cauliflower, mushrooms, yellow squash, red bell pepper, zucchini, carrots and red onions, tomatoes and asparagus.

2.   Stir in the vegetables with olive oil, garlic, balsamic vinegar, thyme, oregano, black pepper and garlic salt

3. Toss the vegetables gently with your hand until they are fully encased with olive oil, herbs, and spices.

4. Spread the seasoned vegetables evenly on a non-stick grilling tray/pan/basket

5. For indirect cooking, set up your wood pellet smoker-grill and preheat it to 425 ° F using any form of wood pellet.

6. To the preheated smoker-grill, transfer the grilling tray and roast the vegetables for 20 to 40 minutes, or until the veggies are al dente. Immediately serve.

3.10 Applewood-Smoked Cheese

Ready in about 3 hours |Servings-Many| Difficulty-Hard

Ingredients

One-to-two and a half-pound block of the following suggested cheeses like

*   Sharp cheddar

*   Gouda

*   Extra-sharp 3-year cheddar

*   Pepper Jack Swiss

*   Monterey Jack

Instructions

1. Break the cheese blocks into compact sizes to maximize smoke penetration based on the form of the cheese blocks.

2. To allow a very thin skin or crust to develop that serves as a barrier to heat but enables the smoke to enter, let the cheese sit uncovered on the counter for 1 hour.

3. Mount a cold-smoke package to customize your wood pellet smoker-grill for indirect fire and plan for cold-smoking.

4. Ensure that the louver vents of the smoker box are completely open to allow the box to avoid moisture.

5. Preheat your smoker-grill wood pellet to 180 ° F, or if you have one, use the smoke mode, using apple pellets for a milder smoke taste.

6. Put the cheese on non-stick grill mats of Teflon-coated fiberglass and cold-smoke for 2 hours.

7. Take the smoked cheese and use a cooling rack to allow it to cool on the counter for an hour.

8. Vacuum-seal and mark your smoked cheeses for a minimum of 2 weeks before refrigerating to enable the smoke to absorb and mellow the cheese's taste.

3.11 Bacon Cheddar Sliders

Ready in 45 minutes | Servings-6 to 10 | Difficulty-Moderate

Ingredients

- Half teaspoon of garlic salt
- Half teaspoon of garlic powder
- Half teaspoon of black pepper
- Half cup of mayonnaise
- Six (1-ounce) slices of sharp cheddar cheese, cut in half
- One and a half pounds ground beef
- Half teaspoon of seasoned salt
- Half teaspoon of onion powder
- Six bacon slices, cut in half

- Two teaspoons of creamy horseradish

- Half small red onion, thinly sliced

- Ketchup

- Half cup of sliced kosher dill pickles12 mini buns

Instructions

1. In a medium dish, blend together the ground beef, seasoned salt, garlic salt, garlic powder, black pepper and onion powder

2. Divide the meat mixture into 12 equal portions and form them into small, thin, circular patties and set aside (approximately 2 ounces each).

3. Over medium pressure, cook the bacon in a medium skillet until crisp, around 5 to 8 minutes. Only put back.

4. Mix the mayonnaise and horseradish, if used, in a wide bowl to render the sauce. In order to use a griddle accessory, customize your wood pellet smoker-grill for direct cooking. Check with your supplier

5. And see if they have a griddle accessory that fits your special smoker-grill for wood pellets.

6. For better non-stick results, coat the griddle's cooking surface with cooking spray.

7. Using the pellets of your choosing, preheat your wood pellet smoker-grill to 350°F. Your griddle's surface should be around 400°F.

8. Grill the patties on either side for 3 to 4 minutes before they are cooked to an internal temperature of 160°F.

9. If needed, put on each patty a slice of sharp cheddar cheese while the patty is still on the griddle or after the patty has been removed from the griddle. On the

bottom half of each roll, put a dollop of the mayonnaise mixture, a red slice of onion, and a burger patty. Pickle slices, sausage, and ketchup on top.

3.12 Teriyaki Steak Bites

Ready in 1 hour and 45 minutes | Servings-4 | Difficulty-Moderate

Ingredients

- Teriyaki Marinade
- One tablespoon of light brown sugar packed
- One teaspoon of garlic salt
- Two pounds of top sirloin steak
- A quarter cup of teriyaki sauce
- One teaspoon of garlic powder
- One tablespoon of soy sauce
- Half teaspoon of pepper
- One tablespoon of apple cider vinegar

Instructions

1.   Mix all of the marinade components together in a tiny mixing bowl.

2.   Trim the steak and split it into 2-inch bits. Place in the Ziploc bag and add in the steak top marinade. Squeeze out as much air as you can and lock the jar. Put in the fridge for a period of 8 hours or overnight.

3.   The steak bites are prepared to be smoked to 225 degrees according to the instructions of the maker until ready to smoke.

4.   Place it on the smoker grates or on a rack right away. Remove the leftover marinade. Smoke for 1 hour and 30 minutes or until 135-140 degrees F is the internal temperature. Remove from the smoker and quickly serve.

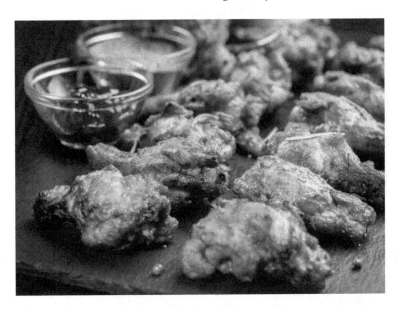

Chapter 4-Lunch Recipes

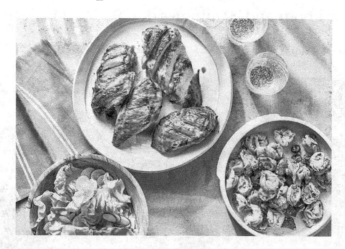

4.1   Jan's Grilled Quarters

Ready in about 2 hours and 15 minutes (marination time excluded) |Servings-4| Difficulty-Hard

Ingredients

- Four fresh or thawed frozen chicken quarters

- Four tablespoons of Jan's Original Dry Rub

- Four to Six tablespoons of extra-virgin olive oil

Instructions

1.   Trim any extra skin and fat off the chicken parts. Peel the chicken skin gently and rub the olive oil on and under each quarter of the chicken skin.

2.   Season with Jan's Initial Dry Rub on and below the skins and on the backs of the chicken parts.

3.   To allow the flavors time to absorb, seal the seasoned chicken pieces in plastic wrap and refrigerate for 2 to 4 hours.

4. Customize your wood pellet smoker-grill for indirect cooking and use some pellets to preheat to 325 ° F.

5. On the barbecue, position the chicken quarters and cook at 325 ° F for 1 hour.

6. To finish the chicken quarters and crisp the skins, lift the pit temperature to 400 ° F after an hour.

7. When the interior temperature, at the thickest areas of the thighs and legs, exceeds 180 ° F, take the crispy chicken quarters off the grill, and the juices flow out.

8. Until eating, rest the grilled spicy chicken quarters under a loose foil tent for 15 minutes.

4.2 Cajun Spatchcock Chicken

Ready in about 3 hours 20 minutes (marination time excluded) |Servings-4| Difficulty-Hard

Ingredients

- Four to five-pound fresh or thawed frozen young chicken
- Four tablespoons of Cajun Spice Rub
- Four to Six tablespoons of extra-virgin olive oil

Instructions

1. Set the breast-side chicken down on a cutting board.

2. In order to extract it, cut down both sides of the backbone using kitchen or poultry shears.

3. To flatten it, turn the chicken over and push tightly down on the breast. Loosen the skin of the breast, thigh, and drumstick gently and peel it down.

4. Apply the olive oil liberally under and on the skin. Season the chicken under the skin on both sides and directly over the flesh.

5.   To allow the flavors time to absorb, cover the chicken in plastic wrap and let it sit for 3 hours in the refrigerator.

6.   For indirect cooking, customize your wood pellet smoker-grill and preheat it to 225°F using hickory, pecan pellets, or a mix.

7.   For an hour and a half, smoke the chicken.

8.   Increase the pit temperature to 375 ° F after one and a half hours at 225 ° F, and roast until the internal temperature at the thickest section of the breast exceeds 170 ° F and the thighs are at least 180 ° F.

9.   Until slicing, rest the chicken under a loose foil tent for 15 minutes.

4.3   Smoked Pork Tenderloins

Ready in about 2 hours (marination time excluded) | Servings-6 | Difficulty-Hard

Ingredients

- Two pork tenderloins (one and a half to two pounds)
- A quarter cup of Jan's Original Dry Rub or Pork Dry Rub
- A quarter cup of roasted garlic–flavored extra-virgin olive oil

Instructions

1.   Trim all of the meat's extra fat and silver skin.

2.   Apply with olive oil and dust both sides of the tenderloins with the rub.3. For 2 to 4 hours, seal the seasoned tenderloins in plastic wrap and refrigerate.

3.   For indirect cooking, set up your wood pellet smoker-grill and preheat it to 230°F utilizing hickory or apple pellets.

4.   Take off the plastic wrap from the meat and place the smoker-grill probes of your wood pellet or a remote meat probe into the thickest section of each tenderloin. If your grill does not have meat probe capability or if you do not have a remote meat

probe, use a wireless instant-read thermometer for internal temperature readings during the cooker.

5.   Set the tenderloins directly on the grill and smoke them at 230 ° F for 45 minutes.

6.   Increase the temperature of the pit to 350 ° F and finish cooking the tenderloins for around 45 more minutes until the interior temperature exceeds 145 ° F at the thickest stage.

7.   Until cooking, rest the pork tenderloins under a thin foil tent for 10 minutes.

4.4   Pellet Grill Smokehouse Burger

Ready in about 1 hour 30 minutes | Servings-6 | Difficulty-Hard

Ingredients

- Two pounds of ground chuck
- One tablespoon of paprika
- One and a half teaspoons of kosher salt
- Six thick-cut bacon slices
- One tablespoon of soy sauce
- One medium-sized red onion
- Six Kaiser rolls
- Six tablespoons ketchup
- A quarter cup of Dijon mustard
- Two teaspoons of onion powder
- One and a half teaspoons of black pepper
- A quarter cup of unsalted butter
- One tablespoon of Worcestershire sauce

PIT BOSS WOOD PELLET GRILL & SMOKER COOKBOOK FOR ATHLETES [4 BOOKS IN 1] BY CHEF MARCELLO RUBY

- Six sharp Cheddar cheese slices

- ¾ cup mayonnaise

- Hickory hardwood pellets

Instructions

1. In compliance with the manufacturer's guidance, fill a pellet jar with hardwood pellets into an electronic pellet grill. Set the temperature of the pellet grill to 415 °F, close the lid and preheat for 10 to 15 minutes.

2. In a big tub, blend the beef, paprika, mustard, garlic powder, onion powder, pepper and salt together. Form into six patties (4-inch-wide).

3. In a broad cast-iron or another heat-resistant pan, place the bacon and place it on the grill grate. Close the lid and grill for 25 to 30 minutes until the bacon is mostly crisp and most of the fat is made. Take the bacon out of the pan and drain it on paper towels. Drain skillet drippings; do not wipe clean skillet.

4. Melt the butter on the grill in a pan. To the skillet, add soy sauce and Worcestershire sauce, then mix to blend. Attach the onions to the skillet and position them on one side of the grill. Place the patties and shut the cover on the other side. Grill before a meat thermometer is placed from 130 ° F to 135 ° F in patty registers, 7 1/2 to 10 minutes per hand. Top the patties with slices of cheese, cover, and barbecue for 1 to 2 minutes before the cheese is melted. Put the buns on the grill, cut side down, and grill for around 1 minute until toasted.

5. Uniformly distributed mayonnaise and ketchup on sliced sides of buns. Place bun bottoms with patties, bacon, and onions; cover with tops, and serve immediately.

4.5   Roasted Leg of Lamb

Ready in about 2 hours 30 minutes (marination time excluded) |Servings-8| Difficulty-Hard

Ingredients

- Half cup of roasted garlic–flavored extra-virgin olive oil

- Three minced garlic cloves

- Two tablespoons of dried oregano

- Half teaspoon of black pepper

- One (Four pounds) boneless leg of lamb

- A quarter cup of dried parsley

- Two tablespoons of fresh-squeezed lemon juice or one tablespoon of lemon zest

- One tablespoon of dried rosemary

Instructions

1.   Remove some netting from the lamb's leg. Trim off any wide bits of gristle, fat, and silver skin.

2.   Mix the olive oil, garlic, parsley, lemon juice or zest, rosemary, oregano and pepper in a shallow dish.

3.   On the inner and outer surfaces of the boneless leg of the lamb, add a spice rub.

4.   To protect the boneless leg of lamb, use silicone food-grade cooking bands or butcher's twine. To build and retain the simple shape of the lamb, use bands or twine.

5.   Cover the lamb loosely with plastic wrap and chill overnight to allow the meat to penetrate the seasonings.

6.   Take the lamb from the fridge and let it stand for an hour at room temperature.

7.   Use the pellets of choice to rig your wood pellet smoker-grill for indirect cooking and preheat it to 400 ° F.

8.   Break the lamb's plastic wrap.

9.   Insert the thickest portion of the lamb with your wood pellet smoker-grill meat probe or a remote meat probe. If your grill does not have meat probe capability or if you do not have a remote meat probe, use a wireless instant-read thermometer for internal temperature readings during the cooker. At 400 °F, roast the lamb until the internal temperature exceeds the ideal doneness at the thickest section.

10.   Until cutting against the grain and cooking, rest the lamb under a loose foil tent for 10 minutes.

4.6   Teriyaki Smoked Drumsticks

Ready in about 2 hours 30 minutes (marination time excluded) |Servings-4| Difficulty-Hard

Ingredients

- Three teaspoons of Poultry Seasoning
- Ten chicken drumsticks
- Three cups of teriyaki marinade and cooking sauce
- One teaspoon of garlic powder

Instructions

1.   Mix the cooking sauce and marinade with the poultry seasoning and garlic powder in a medium bowl.

2.   To facilitate marinade penetration, peel back the skin on the drumsticks.3. Place the drumsticks in a marinating pan or 1-gallon sealable plastic bag and pour over the drumsticks the marinade mixture. Overnight, refrigerate.

3.   Rotate the morning chicken drumsticks.

4.   Configure the indirect cooking of your wood pellet smoker grill.

5.   To drain on a cooking sheet on your counter while the grill is preheating, replace the skin over the drumsticks and hang the drumsticks on a poultry leg-and-wing rack. If you don't own a poultry leg-and-wing rack, you can use paper towels to lightly pat the drumsticks dry.

6.   Using hickory or maple pellets, preheat your wood pellet smoker-grill to 180°F.

7.   Marinated chicken drumsticks should be smoked for 1 hour.

8.   Increase the pit temperature to 350 ° F after an hour and cook the drumsticks for a further 30 to 45 minutes before the interior temperature of the thickest section of the drumsticks exceeds 180 ° F.

9.   Before serving, rest the chicken drumsticks under a loose foil tent for 15 minutes.

4.7   Applewood Walnut-Crusted Rack of Lamb

Ready in about 2 hours (marination time excluded) |Servings-4| Difficulty-Hard

Ingredients

•   Two minced garlic cloves

•   Half teaspoon of kosher salt

- Half teaspoon of rosemary

- One cup of crushed walnuts

- Three tablespoons of Dijon mustard

- Half teaspoon of garlic powder

- Half teaspoon of black pepper

- One rack of lamb (one to two pounds)

Instructions

1. In a small bowl, combine the garlic, mustard, garlic powder, pepper, salt, and rosemary together.

2. Spread evenly on all sides of the lamb with the seasoning mix and sprinkle with the crushed walnuts. To stick the nuts to the meat, press the walnuts lightly with your hand.

3. Wrap the walnut-crusted lamb rack loosely with plastic wrap and cool overnight to allow the meat to penetrate the seasonings.

4. To allow it to reach room temperature, remove the walnut-crusted rack of lamb from the refrigerator and let it relax for 30 minutes.

5. For indirect cooking, configure your wood pellet smoker-grill and preheat it to 225 ° F using apple pellets.

6. Put the bone-side lamb rack down directly on the grill.

7. Smoke at 225 ° F until the thickest part of the lamb rack, measured with a digital instant-read thermometer, reaches the desired internal temperature as you are near the times listed in the chart.

8. Before serving, rest the lamb under a loose foil tent for 5 minutes.

4.8 Hot-Smoked Teriyaki Tuna

Ready in about 9 hours 10 minutes | Servings-4 | Difficulty-Hard

Ingredients

- Two cups of Mr. Yoshida's Traditional Teriyaki Marinade and Cooking Sauce
- Two (10-ounce) fresh tuna steaks

Instructions

1. Slice the tuna into slices that are uniformly thick, about 2 inches thick.

2. Place the tuna slices along with the marinade in a 1-gallon sealable plastic bag and place it in a shallow baking dish in case of a leak. Let the tuna rotate every hour and sit in the refrigerator for 3 hours.

3. Remove the tuna from the marinade after 3 hours and lightly pat it dry with a paper towel.

4. Enable the tuna to air-dry for 2 to 4 hours in the refrigerator, uncovered, until pellicles form.

5. For indirect cooking, configure your wood pellet smoker-grill and preheat it to 180 ° F using alder pellets.

6. On a Teflon-coated fiberglass mat or directly on the grill grates, place the tuna pieces, and smoke the tuna for an hour.

7. Increase the temperature of the pit to 250°F after 1 hour. Cook for another 1 hour until the internal temperature reaches 145 degrees F.

8. Remove the tuna from the grill and leave to rest before serving for 10 minutes.

4.9 Baked Fresh Wild Sockeye Salmon

Ready in about 40 minutes | Servings-6 | Difficulty-Moderate

Ingredients

- Two fresh wild sockeye salmon fillets
- 3⁄4 teaspoon of Old Bay seasoning
- Two teaspoons of Seafood Seasoning

Instructions

1. Rinse the salmon fillets with cool water and wipe them dry with a paper towel.

2. Lightly brush the fillets with the seasonings.

3. Customize your wood pellet smoker-grill for indirect cooking and preheat to 400°F using some pellets.

4. Lay the skin-side down of salmon on a Teflon-coated fiberglass mat or directly on the grill grates.

5. Bake the salmon for 15 to 20 minutes before the internal temperature exceeds 140°F, and/or the meat flakes easily with a fork.

6. Rest the salmon for 5 minutes before eating.

4.10 Bacon Cordon Bleu

Ready in about 3 hours 15 minutes | Servings-6 | Difficulty-Hard

Ingredients

- Three large skinless and butterflied boneless chicken breasts
- Three tablespoons of Jan's Original Dry Rub or Poultry Seasoning
- Twelve slices of provolone cheese
- Twenty-four bacon slices
- Three tablespoons of roasted garlic–flavored extra-virgin olive oil

- Twelve slices of black forest ham

Instructions

1. Weave four bacon slices closely together, leaving extra room at the ends. Alternate bacon slices are interlocked by the bacon weave and used to wind around the chicken cordon bleu.

2. Spritz or brush two thin chicken breast fillets on both sides with olive oil.

3. With the seasoning, clean all sides of the chicken breast fillets.

4. On the bacon weave, plate one seasoned chicken fillet and finish with one slice of each ham and Provolone cheese.

5. Using another chicken fillet, ham, and cheese, repeat the operation. Fold in half the chicken, ham and cheese.

6. To cover the chicken cordon blue fully, overlap the bacon strips from opposite ends.

7. To keep the bacon strips in place, use silicone food-grade cooking bands, butcher's twine, or toothpicks.

8. For the leftover chicken breasts and ingredients, repeat the procedure.

9. Configure your wood pellet smoker-grill with apple or cherry pellets for indirect cooking and preheating for smoking (180 ° F to 200 ° F).

10. For 1 hour, smoke the bacon cordon bleu.

11. Increase the pit temperature to 350°F after smoking for an hour.

12. If the internal temperature exceeds 165 ° F and the bacon is crisp, the bacon cordon bleu is cooked.

13. Until eating, rest under a loose foil tent for 15 minutes.

4.11 Pulled Hickory-smoked Pork Butts

Ready in about 11 hours (marination time excluded) |Servings-20 or more| Difficulty-Hard

Ingredients

- Two (10-pound) boneless pork butts, vacuum-packed or fresh

- 3⁄4 cup of Pork Dry Rub, Jan's Original Dry Rub or your favorite pork rub

- One cup of roasted garlic–flavored extra-virgin olive oil

Instructions

1. If you see fit, take off the fat cap and any readily accessible broad portions of surplus fat from each pork ass. Some tend to reduce the fat cap to a quarter of an inch or keep the whole fat cap on because they assume that when they roast, the melting fat bastes the butts. In areas protected by fat, this process prevents the development of bark.

2. Break each butt of pork in half. To keep the meat intact through cooking and handling, use silicone food-grade cooking bands or butcher's twine.

3. Rub the oil over all the sides of each pork ass. Sprinkle a liberal sum of the rub with each pork butt and pat it with your fist.

4. The seasoned boneless pork butts are individually double-wrapped in plastic wrap and refrigerated overnight.

5. For indirect cooking, set up your wood pellet smoker-grill and preheat it to 225 ° F utilizing hickory pellets.

6. Takedown the pork butts from the refrigerator and, when preheating your wood pellet smoker-grill, remove the plastic wrap.

7.   There's no need for pork butts to totally hit room temperature. In the thickest section of one or more pork butts, place your wood pellet smoker-grill meat probes or a remote meat probe. If your grill does not have meat probe capability or you do not possess a remote meat probe, for internal temperature measurements, use an instant-read wireless thermometer during the cook.3. Smoke the butts of pork for 3 hours.

8.   Increase the pit temperature to 350 °F after 3 hours and cook before the butts' internal temperature exceeds 160 °F.

9.   Take the butts of pork from the barbecue and cover each one in heavy-duty aluminum foil twice. Take caution to ensure that when you double-wrap them, you hold the meat probes in the butts.

10.   To your 350°F pellet smoker-grill, return the wrapped pork butts.

11.   Until the internal temperature of the pork butts exceeds 200 ° to 205 ° F, continue cooking the foil-wrapped pork butts.

12.   Prior to pulling and cooking, remove the pork butts and FTC for 3 to 4 hours.

13.   Using your preferred pulling tool, pull the smoked pork butts into little succulent shreds.

14.   Mix the pulled pork butts with any remaining liquid if you'd like. On a fresh-baked roll topped with coleslaw, serve the pulled pork with barbecue sauce or serve the pulled pork with condiments such as lettuce, tomato, red onion, mayo, horseradish and cheese.

4.12   Pellet Grill Pork Loin with Salsa Verde

Ready in about 1 hour 15 minutes | Servings-8 | Difficulty-Hard

Ingredients

Salsa Verde

- Half cup of finely chopped shallots

- ⅓ cup chopped fresh cilantro

- One tablespoon of chopped capers

- One teaspoon of grated garlic

- One teaspoon of kosher salt

- Four chopped anchovy fillets

- One cup of olive oil

- ⅓ cup of chopped fresh flat-leaf parsley

- A quarter cup of chopped fresh dill

- One teaspoon of grated lemon zest

- One teaspoon of grated fresh ginger

- ¾ teaspoon crushed red pepper

Pork Loin

- Two teaspoons of kosher salt

- Three tablespoons of fresh lemon juice

- Three and a half pounds boneless

- One teaspoon of black pepper

Instructions

1. Prepare Salsa Verde: In a medium dish, stir together all the ingredients. Just set aside.

2. Prepare the Pork Loin: Fill a pellet jar with hardwood pellets on an electric pellet grill as instructed by the maker. Set the temperature of the pellet grill to 350

°F, close the lid and preheat for 10 to 15 minutes. Sprinkle the pork with salt and pepper all around.

3. Place the pork on the grill, close the lid, and grill on both sides until lightly browned, about 7 1/2 minutes per side. Spin the pork up with the fat cap if necessary, and finish with half the Salsa Verde. Cover the lid and barbecue for 25 to 30 minutes before a meat thermometer inserted into the thickest part registers 140 ° F.

4. Take the pork off the grill and let it sit for 15 minutes before slicing. Mix the lemon juice and the remaining Salsa Verde together, and spoon over the sliced pork.

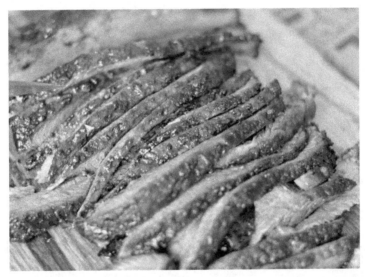

Chapter 5-Dinner Recipes

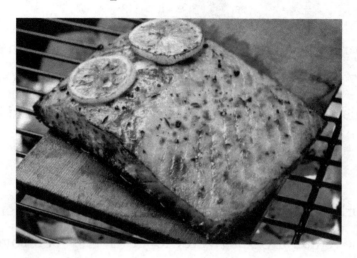

5.1   Roasted Tuscan Thighs

Ready in about 1 hour and 45 minutes (marination time excluded) | Servings-4 | Difficulty-Hard

Ingredients

- Eight chicken thighs
- Three teaspoons of Tuscan Seasoning or any Tuscan seasoning, per thigh
- Three tablespoons of roasted garlic–flavored extra-virgin olive oil

Instructions

1.   Trim any extra skin from the chicken thighs to prepare for shrinkage, preserving a quarter of an inch.

2.   Peel back the skin gently to clear any large fat deposits under the skin and on the back of the leg.

3.   Apply the olive oil gently on and under the skin and back of the thighs. Season with Tuscan seasoning on and below the surface and back of the thighs.

4.   To allow the flavors time to absorb before roasting, seal the chicken thighs in plastic wrap and refrigerate for 1 to 2 hours.

5.   Configure your wood pellet smoker-grill for indirect cooking and use some pellets to preheat to 375 ° F.

6.   Roast the chicken thighs for 40 to 60 minutes, depending on your wood pellet smoker-grill, before the internal temperature at the thickest section of the thighs exceeds 180 ° F. Until eating, rest the roasted Tuscan thighs under a loose foil tent for 15 minutes.

5.2   Smoked Bone-In Turkey Breast

Ready in about 5 hours | Servings-6 to 8 | Difficulty-Hard

Ingredients

*   One (eight to ten pound) bone-in turkey breast
*   Five tablespoons of Jan's Original Dry Rub or Poultry Seasoning
*   Six tablespoons of extra-virgin olive oil

Instructions

1.   Trim away some extra turkey breast fat and skin.

2.   Separate the skin from the breast cautiously, keeping the skin preserved. Within the breast hollow, under the skin and on the skin, apply the olive oil.

3.   Season the breast cavity generously with rub or seasoning, under the surface, and on the skin.

4.   Place the turkey breast, breast-side up, in a V-rack for better handling or directly on the grill grates.

5.   Enable the turkey breast on your kitchen countertop to rest at room temperature when preheating your wood pellet smoker barbecue.

6.   For indirect cooking, set your wood pellet smoker-grill and preheat it to 225°F utilizing hickory or pecan pellets.

7.   For 2 hours, smoke the bone-in turkey breast at 225 °F on the V-rack or directly on the grill grates.

8.   Elevate the temperature of the pit to 325 ° F after 2 hours of hickory smoke. Roast until an internal temperature of 170 ° F hits the thickest section of the turkey breast, and the juices run clear.

9.   Before cutting against the grain, rest the hickory-smoked turkey breast under a loose foil tent for 20 minutes.

5.3   Crab-Stuffed Lemon Cornish Hens

Ready in about 2 hours 15 minutes (marination time excluded) |Servings-2 to 4| Difficulty-Hard

Ingredients

- Two Cornish hens
- Four tablespoons of Pete's Western Rub or any poultry rub
- One halved lemon
- Two cups of Crabmeat Stuffing

Instructions

1.   Rinse the hens inside and out vigorously and pat off. Loosen the breast and leg skin cautiously. Under and on the skin and inside the cavity, rub the lemon. Rub the Western Pete's Rub under and on the skin of the breast and thigh. Return the skin to its original location cautiously.

2.   To allow the flavors time to mature, seal the Cornish hens in plastic wrap and refrigerate for 2 to 3 hours.

3.   Prepare according to the guidelines for the Crabmeat Stuffing. Before stuffing the hens, make sure it has cooled absolutely. Stuff each hen cavity loosely with the crab stuffing.

4.   To hold the stuffing in, bind the Cornish hen legs together with butcher's twine.

5.   Set your wood pellet smoker-grill with some pellets for indirect cooking and preheat to 375 ° F.

6.   Place the stuffed hens inside a baking dish on a shelf. If you don't have a rack small enough to match, you may also directly position the hens in the baking bowl.

7.   The hens are roasted at 375 ° F until the internal temperature exceeds 170 ° F at the thickest section of the breast, the thighs exceed 180 ° F, and the juices run clear.

8.   To see if it has hit a temperature of 165°F, measure the crabmeat stuffing.

9.   Until eating, rest the roasted hens under a loose foil tent for 15 minutes.

5.4   Double-Smoked Ham

Ready in about 2 hours | Servings-8 to 12 | Difficulty-Hard

Ingredients

•   One (ten pounds) applewood-smoked, boneless, fully cooked, ready-to-eat ham or bone-in smoked ham

Instructions

1.   Take the ham from its wrapping and allow to rest for 30 minutes at room temperature.

2.   Depending on what kind of wood was used for the initial smoking, customize your wood pellet smoker-grill for indirect cooking and preheat it to 180°F using apple or hickory pellets.

3.   Directly put the ham on the grill grates and smoke the ham at 180°F for 1 hour.

4.   Elevate the pit temperature to 350 ° F after an hour.

5.   Cook the ham for around one and a half to 2 more hours before the internal temperature exceeds 140 ° F.

6.   Until cutting against the grain, cut the ham and cover it in foil for 15 minutes.

5.5   Easy No-Fail Pellet Smoker Ribs

Ready in about 6 hours | Servings-4 | Difficulty-Hard

Ingredients

- Two racks of Baby Back or Spare Ribs
- BBQ Rib Rub

Instructions

1.   Begin preheating your pellet smoker at 225 degrees F as you are prepping the ribs. Following the directions and start-up procedure of your pellet smoker brand is critical.

2.   Ribs normally come on the underside of the rack with a thin coat of rough muscle. This is known as the silver skin, and it has to be extracted so that the meat can penetrate the seasonings.

3.   On a sheet tray, put the ribs and apply around 2-3 tablespoons of rib rub each hand. You don't want to coat them fully to make any of the meat peek in.

4.   You may position the rack (or two racks) directly on the grates until the smoker is preheated and let them burn. Leave them for at least 4 hours alone. The shorter you open your barbecue, the shorter your cooking period would be. You

ought to keep an eye on the temperature of the smoker to ensure it remains where it is placed.

5.   It will take 4 or 5 hours for a rack of baby back ribs to cook, and it will take 6 to 7 hours for spare ribs.

6.   Pick up the ribs with tongs at the end of the cooking time, and if the bark splits and the ribs are nearly cut in two, they are cooked. Keep on smoking if not.

7.   Add sauce to the BBQ. You should cover them with a thin film of your preferred BBQ sauce when the ribs are about to come out of the smoker (they passed the bending test). For 30 more minutes, keep them on the smoker at 225 degrees F so that the sauce will caramelize.

5.6   Texas-Style Brisket Flat

Ready in about 10 hours 45 minutes | Servings-8 to 10 | Difficulty-Hard

Ingredients

- Six and a Half pound beef brisket flat
- Half cup of Texas-Style Brisket Rub or your favorite brisket rub
- Half cup of roasted garlic–flavored extra-virgin olive oil

Instructions

1.   Trim the brisket's fat cap off and extract any silver skin.2. Rub the trimmed meat with olive oil on both ends.

2.   Apply the rub on both sides of the brisket, making sure that the rub is thoroughly coated.

3.   Double-cover the brisket in plastic wrap and refrigerate overnight to reach the beef with the rub, or you can quickly sear the brisket if you choose.

4.   Take the brisket from the fridge and put the smoker-grill wood pellet or a remote meat probe into the thickest portion of the meat. If you don't have a meat probe, capabilities or a remote meat probe on your barbecue, then use an instant-read optical thermometer for internal temperature readings during the cooker.

5.   For indirect cooking, set up your wood pellet smoker-grill and preheat it to 250 ° F using mesquite or oak pellets.

6.   At 250°F, smoke the brisket before the inner temperature exceeds 160°F (about 4 hours).

7.   Remove the grill from the brisket, double-wrap it in heavy-duty aluminum foil, make sure the meat probe is left in place, and add it to the grill for smokers.

8.   Increase the temperature of the pit to 325 ° F, then cook the brisket for another 2 hours before the internal temperature exceeds 205 ° F.

9.   The foiled brisket is cut, wrapped in a cloth, and put in a cooler. Let sit 2 to 4 hours in the cooler before slicing against the grain and serving.

5.7   Hickory-Smoked Prime Rib of Pork

Ready in about 4 hours 15 minutes (marination time excluded) |Servings-6| Difficulty-Hard

Ingredients

- One (Five pounds) rack of pork, about six ribs

- Six tablespoons of Jan's Original Dry Rub, Pork Dry Rub or your favorite pork roast rub

- A quarter cup of roasted garlic–flavored extra-virgin olive oil

Instructions

1.   Trim the fat cap and silver skin off the pork rack. A rack of pork has a membrane on the bones, much like a slice of ribs. Using a spoon handle under the bone membrane to loosen the membrane from the bones so you can reach the membrane with a paper towel to take it off.

2.   On both sides of the beef, rub the olive oil liberally. Season with the seasoning, coating the beef on both sides. 3. The seasoned rack of pork is double covered in plastic wrap and refrigerated for 2 to 4 hours or overnight.

3.   Take the seasoned pork rack from the refrigerator and let it rest for 30 minutes before cooking at room temperature.

4.   For indirect cooking, set up your wood pellet smoker-grill and preheat it to 225 ° F utilizing hickory pellets.

5.   Insert into the thickest portion of the rack of pork the wood pellet smoker-grill meat probe or a remote meat probe. Using an instant-read wireless thermometer while cooking for internal temperature readings if your grill does not have meat probe capability or you do not have a remote meat probe.

6.   Set the rib-side of the rack down directly on the grill grates.

7.   For 3 to 3 and a half hours, smoke the pork rack before the internal temperature exceeds 140 ° F.

8.   Remove from the smoker's meat and let it rest 15 minutes before being carved under a loose foil tent.

5.8   Meaty Chuck Short Ribs

Ready in about 6 hours 35 minutes | Servings- 2 to 4 | Difficulty-Hard

Ingredients

- English-cut 4-bone slab beef chuck short ribs

- Three to five tablespoons of Pete's Western Rub
- Three to four tablespoons of yellow mustard or extra-virgin olive oil

Instructions

1. Remove some silver skin by trimming the fat cap off the ribs, leaving a quarter of an inch of fat.

2. To season the meat correctly by working a spoon handle under the membrane to get a slice raised, separate the membrane from the bones. To catch the membrane, use a paper towel to take it off the bones.

3. Slather both sides of the short rib slab with mustard or olive oil. With the rub, season liberally on both edges.

4. Using mesquite or hickory pellets, set up your wood pellet smoker-grill for indirect heat and preheat to 225 ° F.

5. In the thickest section of the slab of ribs, place your wood pellet smoker-grill or a remote meat probe. If your grill does not have meat probe capability or you do not have a remote meat probe, then for internal temperature measurements, use an instant-read optical thermometer during the cooker.

6. On the grill, put the short ribs bone-side down and smoke for 5 hours at 225 ° F.

7. If the ribs have not achieved an internal temperature of at least 195 ° F after 5 hours, so the pit temperature can rise to 250 ° F before the inner temperature exceeds 195 °F to 205 ° F.

8. Until eating, rest the smoked short ribs under a loose foil tent for 15 minutes.

5.9   Roasted Duck à I' Orange

Ready in about 3 hours and 50 minutes | Servings-3 to 4 | Difficulty-Hard

Ingredients

- One (Five to six-pound) frozen Long Island, Peking, or Canadian duck

- One large orange, cut into wedges

- Half small red onion, quartered

- Three tablespoons of Pete's Western Rub or Poultry Seasoning, divided

- Three celery stalks, chopped into large chunks

For the sauce

- Two cups of orange juice

- Two tablespoons of orange marmalade

- Three teaspoons of grated fresh ginger

- Two tablespoons of soy sauce

- Two tablespoons of honey

Instructions

1.   Remove any giblets from the duck's cavity and neck and keep or dispose of them for some purpose. With a paper towel, clean the duck and pat it off.

2.   From the tail, spine, and cavity section, trim any extra fat. Using the tip of a sharp paring knife to poke the duck skin all over to make sure that it does not reach the duck meat to promote the removal of the fat layer under the flesh.

3.   With one tablespoon of rub or seasoning, season the interior of the cavity.

4.   With the remaining rub or seasoning, season the outside of the duck.

5.   Stuff the space with orange wedges, celery, and onion. To aid hold the stuffing in, bind the duck legs together with butcher's twine. On a small rack in a shallow roasting pan, put the duck breast-side up.

6. Mix the ingredients in a saucepan over low heat to create the sauce and boil until the sauce thickens and is syrupy.

7. Enable to cool and put aside.

8. Set up your wood pellet smoker-grill for indirect cooking and use some pellets to preheat it to 350 ° F.

9. Roast the duck for 2 hours at 350°F.

10. Brush the duck liberally with the orange sauce after 2 hours.

11. Roast the orange-glazed duck for another 30 minutes and check that the internal temperature exceeds 165 °F at the thickest section of the legs.

12. Until cooking, rest the duck under a loose foil tent for 20 minutes.

13. Throw out the orange wedges, onion and celery. Quarter the duck with shears of poultry and serve.

5.10   Peteizza Meatloaf

Ready in about 3 hours 30 minutes | Servings-8 | Difficulty-Hard

Ingredients

For meatloaf

- Two large eggs
- One cup of Italian bread crumbs
- Half teaspoon of seasoned salt
- One pound pork sausage
- One pound ground beef
- Half teaspoon of garlic salt
- Half teaspoon of ground pepper
- Half teaspoon of granulated garlic

- Half cup of pizza sauce, plus an additional half cup for serving

For stuffing

- Two tablespoons of extra-virgin olive oil

- 2/3 cup of sliced green bell pepper

- A pinch of salt and black pepper

- Three ounces of sliced pepperoni sausage

- One cup of sliced portobello mushrooms

- 2/3 cup of sliced red onion

- Half cup of sliced red bell pepper

- Two cups of shredded mozzarella cheese

- Two cups of shredded cheddar or Jack cheese

Instructions

1. Combine the meatloaf components thoroughly with your hands in a wide bowl to achieve maximum performance.

2. Heat the olive oil over medium-high heat in a medium skillet and sauté the mushrooms, green bell pepper, red onion and red bell pepper until the vegetables are al dente for about 2 minutes. With a pinch of salt and black pepper, season the vegetables. Then set it aside.

3. Flatten the meatloaf into a 3/8-inch-thick rectangle on parchment paper. Range the sautéed vegetables thinly over the meat. Cover the mozzarella with the veggies, accompanied by the cheddar or Jack. Cover the pepperoni with the cheese.

4. Using the parchment paper to roll the meatloaf, ensuring the ends and all seams are covered.

5. Set up your wood pellet-smoker grill for indirect heat and use oak pellets or a mix to preheat it to 225 ° F.

6. Smoke a meatloaf with stuffed pizza for 1 hour.

7. Increase the pit temperature to 350 °F after an hour, and cook until the stuffed pizza meatloaf's internal temperature exceeds 170 °F.

8. Cover the meatloaf with the leftover half cup of pizza sauce and allow to stand for 15 minutes under a loose foiled tent before eating.

5.11   Shrimp-Stuffed Tilapia

Ready in about 1 hour 10 minutes | Servings-5 | Difficulty-Moderate

Ingredients

- Two tablespoons of extra-virgin olive oil

- One and a half teaspoons of Seafood Seasoning or Old Bay seasoning

- Five (four to six-ounce) fresh farmed tilapia fillets

- One and a half teaspoons of smoked paprika

For the shrimp Stuffing

- One tablespoon of salted butter

- One cup of Italian bread crumbs

- One large egg, beaten

- One and a half teaspoons of Fagundes Famous Seasoning or salt and pepper

- One pound of cooked, peeled, deveined, tail-off shrimp

- One cup of finely diced red onion

- Half cup of mayonnaise

- Two teaspoons of fresh chopped parsley or dried parsley

Instructions

1.   Get the shrimp stuffing packed. To cut the shrimp finely, use a food processor, salsa maker, or knife.

2.   Melt the butter and sauté the red onion in a small skillet over medium-high heat until it is translucent around 3 minutes. Put aside to let the room temperature cool.

3.   In a wide cup, mix the shrimp, the cooled sautéed onion and the remaining ingredients.

4.   Cover the shrimp stuffing and refrigerate it before ready to use. Shrimp stuffing can be used within two days.

5.   With olive oil, rub all sides of the fillets.

6.   On the backside of each filet, spoon 1/3 cup of the stuffing. Reddish stripping is on the backside of the tilapia fillet.

7.   On the lower half of the fillet, flatten out the stuffing. Fold the tilapia in half and make careful to keep the fish in place with two or more toothpicks.

8.   With the smoked paprika and seafood seasoning or Old Bay seasoning, dust each fillet.

9.   Configure your wood pellet smoker-grill for indirect cooking and use any pellets to preheat it to 400 °F.

10.   On a nonstick grilling tray, position the stuffed fillets.

11.   Bake the tilapia for 30 to 45 minutes, or until the fish quickly flakes and hits an internal temperature of 145°F.

12.   Rest the fish for 5 minutes before serving.

5.12   Easy Smoked Chicken Breasts

Ready in about 45 minutes | Servings-4 | Difficulty-Moderate

Ingredients

- One tablespoon of Olive Oil

- Two tablespoons of Turbinado Sugar

- Two tablespoons of Paprika

- One teaspoon of Black Pepper

- Two tablespoons of garlic powder

- Four Skinless Chicken Breasts Large Boneless

- Two tablespoons of Brown sugar

- One teaspoon of Celery Seed

- Two tablespoons of Kosher salt

- One teaspoon of Cayenne Pepper

- Two tablespoons onion powder

Instructions

1. Mix all the dried ingredients together in a tub.

2. On both sides, pat the chicken breasts to dry and drizzle each side with a little olive oil.

3. Sprinkle the rub liberally on top of the chicken breasts. Enable 15 minutes, or up to 30 minutes, to sit in the fridge (place plastic wrap over the top if over 15 minutes of rest time.)

4. Hot a cigarette smoker (use the super smoke on Traeger) with the lid opened for 5 minutes. Increase the heat to 350 degrees and, as it warms up, shut the cover for 15 minutes.

5. Place the chicken on the grill, spiced side down, and season the underside of the chicken liberally. Cook with the lid closed for 12-13 minutes.

6. Switch over the chicken and cook at 165-170 degrees for another 10-12 minutes or until finished.

7. Take the chicken from the grill and lay a cutting board with foil over the end. Prior to slicing, let the chicken rest for 3-5 minutes.

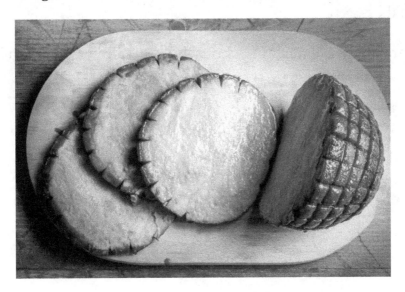

Conclusion

To conclude, the wood pellet smoker grill is scrumptious, pleasant and clean, unmatched by barbecue or gas grills. The smoke composition is milder than you may be accustomed to from other cigarettes. They produce the flexibility and advantages of a convection oven due to their architecture. Smoker-grills with wood pellets is safe and easy to work.

In the 1990s, wood pellet smoker-grills were first launched by a small business named Traeger Grills in Oregon.

Only after Traeger's initial patent expired did the business expand by leaps and bounds. More and more people have been introduced to the amazing, mouth-watering food from a wood pellet smoker-grill, but only two firms created wood pellet smoker-grills as recently as 2008: Traeger and its competitor MAK, both located in Oregon. Currently, a wide variety of retailers from small BBQ stores, grocery stores, produce stores, hardware stores, huge box stores, online outlets, and direct from the retailer hold more than twenty brands of incredible wood pellet smoker-grill makers.

In the present era, it is a must in every household that loves to have a barbeque meal at weekends.

This book is a guide that provides us with information regarding the wood pellet smoker grill and provides the recipes for starting up with grilling.

We hope that all your queries are clear with regards to wood Pellet Smoker Grill cooking.

Thank you and good luck!

Air Fryer Cookbook for Two

Cook and Taste Tens of Healthy Fried Recipes with Your Sweetheart. Burn Fat, Kill Hunger, and Improve Your Mood

By

Chef Marcello Ruby

Table of Contents

INTRODUCTION: 316

CHAPTER 1: AIR FRYER BREAKFAST RECIPES 321

   1. AIR FRYER BREAKFAST FRITTATA 321

   2. AIR FRYER BANANA BREAD 322

   3. EASY AIR FRYER OMELET 324

   4. AIR-FRIED BREAKFAST BOMBS 325

   5. AIR FRYER FRENCH TOAST 326

   6. BREAKFAST POTATOES IN THE AIR FRYER 328

   7. AIR FRYER BREAKFAST POCKETS 329

   8. AIR FRYER SAUSAGE BREAKFAST CASSEROLE 331

   9. BREAKFAST EGG ROLLS 333

   10. AIR FRYER BREAKFAST CASSEROLE 336

   11. AIR FRYER BREAKFAST SAUSAGE INGREDIENTS 338

   12. WAKE UP AIR FRYER AVOCADO BOATS 338

   12. AIR FRYER CINNAMON ROLLS 340

   13. AIR-FRYER ALL-AMERICAN BREAKFAST DUMPLINGS 341

CHAPTER 2: AIR FRYER SEAFOOD RECIPE 343

   1. AIR FRYER 'SHRIMP BOIL' 343

   2. AIR FRYER FISH & CHIPS 344

   3. AIR-FRYER SCALLOPS 345

   4. AIR FRYER TILAPIA 346

   5. AIR FRYER SALMON 348

   6. BLACKENED FISH TACOS IN THE AIR FRYER 350

   7. AIR FRYER COD 352

   8. AIR FRYER MISO-GLAZED CHILEAN SEA BASS 354

   9. AIR FRYER FISH TACOS 357

   10. AIR FRYER SOUTHERN FRIED CATFISH 359

   11. AIR FRYER LOBSTER TAILS WITH LEMON BUTTER 361

   12. AIR FRYER CRAB CAKES WITH SPICY AIOLI + LEMON VINAIGRETTE 363

CHAPTER 3: AIR FRYER MEAT AND BEEF RECIPE 366

   1. AIR FRYER STEAK 366

   2. AIR-FRYER GROUND BEEF WELLINGTON 367

   3. AIR-FRIED BURGERS 368

4. AIR FRYER MEATLOAF 370

5. AIR FRYER HAMBURGERS 372

6. AIR FRYER MEATLOAF 375

7. AIR FRYER BEEF KABOBS... 376

8. AIR-FRIED BEEF AND VEGETABLE SKEWERS 377

9. AIR FRYER TACO CALZONES 379

10. AIR FRYER POT ROAST 380

CHAPTER 4: MIDNIGHT SNACKS.. 382

1. AIR FRYER ONION RINGS 382

2. AIR FRYER SWEET POTATO CHIPS 383

3. AIR FRYER TORTILLA CHIPS 384

4. AIR FRYER ZESTY CHICKEN WINGS 385

5. AIR FRYER SWEET POTATO FRIES 386

6. AIR FRYER CHURROS WITH CHOCOLATE SAUCE............................. 386

7. WHOLE-WHEAT PIZZAS IN AN AIR FRYER 388

8. AIR-FRIED CORN DOG BITES.. 389

9. CRISPY VEGGIE QUESADILLAS IN AN AIR FRYER 390

10. AIR-FRIED CURRY CHICKPEAS 393

11. AIR FRY SHRIMP SPRING ROLLS WITH SWEET CHILI SAUCE............ 394

CHAPTER 5: DESSERT RECIPES 396

1. AIR FRYER MORES.. 396

2. EASY AIR FRYER BROWNIES 397

3. EASY AIR FRYER CHURROS.. 398

4. AIR FRYER SWEET APPLES 400

5. AIR FRYER PEAR CRISP FOR TWO 401

6. KETO CHOCOLATE CAKE – AIR FRYER RECIPE 402

CONCLUSION: 404

Introduction:

You have got the set of important knives, toaster oven, coffee machine, and quick pot along with the cutter you want to good care of. There may be a variety of things inside your kitchen, but maybe you wish to make more space for an air fryer. It's easy to crowd and load with the new cooking equipment even though you've a lot of them. However, an air fryer is something you will want to make space for.

The air fryer is identical to the oven in the way that it roasts and bakes, but the distinction is that elements of hating are placed over the top& are supported by a big, strong fan, producing food that is extremely crispy and, most importantly with little oil in comparison to the counterparts which are deeply fried. Usually, air fryers heat up pretty fast and, because of the centralized heat source & the fan size and placement, they prepare meals quickly & uniformly. The cleanup is another huge component of the air frying. Many baskets & racks for air fryers are dishwasher protected. We recommend a decent dish brush for those who are not dishwasher secure. It will go through all the crannies and nooks that facilitate the movement of air without making you crazy.

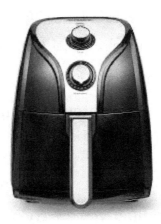

We have seen many rave reviews of this new trend, air frying. Since air frying, they argue, calls for fast and nutritious foods. But is the hype worth it? How do the air fryers work? Does it really fry food?

How do air fryers work?

First, let's consider how air fryer really works before we go to which type of air fryer is decent or any simple recipes. Just think of it; cooking stuff without oil is such a miracle. Then, how could this even be possible? Let's try to find out how to pick the best air fryer for your use now when you understand how the air fryer works.

How to pick the best air fryer

It is common to get lost when purchasing gadgets & electrical equipment, given that there're a wide range of choices available on the market. So, before investing in one, it is really ideal to have in mind the specifications and budget.

Before purchasing the air fryer, you can see the things you should consider:

Capacity/size: Air fryers are of various sizes, from one liter to sixteen liters. A three-liter capacity is fine enough for bachelors. Choose an air fryer that has a range of 4–6 liters for a family having two children. There is a restricted size of the basket which is used to put the food. You will have to prepare the meals in batches if you probably wind up using a tiny air fryer.

Timer: Standard air fryers arrive with a range timer of 30 minutes. For house cooking, it is satisfactory. Thought, if you are trying complex recipes which take a longer cooking time, pick the air fryer with a 1-hour timer.

Temperature: The optimum temperature for most common air fryers is 200 degrees C (400 f). You can quickly prepare meat dishes such as fried chicken, tandoori, kebabs etc.

The design, durability, brand value and controls are other considerations you might consider.

Now that you know which air fryer is best for you let's see the advantages of having an air fryer at your place.

What are the benefits of air fryers?

The benefits of air fryers are as follows:

Cooking with lower fat & will promote weight loss

Air fryers work with no oils and contain up to 80 percent lower fat than most fryers relative to a traditional deep fryer. Shifting to an air fryer may encourage loss of weight by decreasing fat & caloric intake for anyone who consumes fried food regularly and also has a problem with leaving the fast foods.

Faster time for cooking

Air frying is easier comparing with other cooking techniques, such as grilling or baking. Few air fryers need a preheat of 60 seconds, but others do not need a preheat any longer than a grill or an oven. So if there is a greater capacity or multiple compartments for the air fryer basket, you may make various dishes in one go.

Quick to clean

It's extremely easy to clean an air fryer. And after each use, air frying usually does not create enough of a mess except you cook fatty food such as steak or chicken wings. Take the air fryer out and clean it with soap & water in order to disinfect the air fryer.

Safer to be used

The air fryer is having no drawbacks, unlike hot plates or deep frying. Air fryers get hot, but splashing or spilling is not a risk.

Minimum use of electricity and environment friendly

Air fryers consume far less electricity than various electric ovens, saving your money & reducing carbon output.

Flexibility

Some of the air fryers are multi-functional. It's possible to heat, roast, steam, broil, fry or grill food.

Less waste and mess

Pan-fries or deep fryer strategies leave one with excess cooking oil, which is difficult to rid of and usually unsustainable. You can cook fully oil-less food with an air fryer. All the pieces have a coating of nonstick, dishwasher safe and nonstick coating.

Cooking without the use of hands

The air fryer includes a timer, & when it is full, it'll stop by itself so that you may feel secure while multitasking.

Feasible to use

It is very much convenient; you can use an air fryer whenever you want to. Few air fryers involve preheating, which is less than 5 minutes; with the air fryer, one may begin cooking immediately.

Reducing the possibility of the development of toxic acrylamide

Compared to making food in oil, air frying will decrease the potential of producing acrylamides. Acrylamide is a compound that, under elevated temperature cooking, appears in certain food and may have health impacts.

Chapter 1: Air fryer breakfast recipes

96. 1. Air fryer breakfast frittata

Cook time: 20 minutes

Servings: 2 people

Difficulty: Easy

Ingredients:

- 1 pinch of cayenne pepper (not necessary)

- 1 chopped green onion

- Cooking spray

- 2 tbsp. diced red bell pepper

- ¼ pound fully cooked and crumbled breakfast sausages

- 4 lightly beaten eggs

- ½ cup shredded cheddar-Monterey jack cheese blend

Instructions:

1. Combine eggs, bell pepper, cheddar Monterey Jack cheese, sausages, cayenne and onion inside a bowl & blend to combine.

2. The air fryer should be preheated to 360 ° f (180° c). Spray a 6 by 2-inch non-stick cake pan along with a spray used in cooking.

3. Place the mixture of egg in the ready-made cake tray.

4. Cook for 18 - 20 minutes in your air fryer before the frittata is ready.

97. 2. Air fryer banana bread

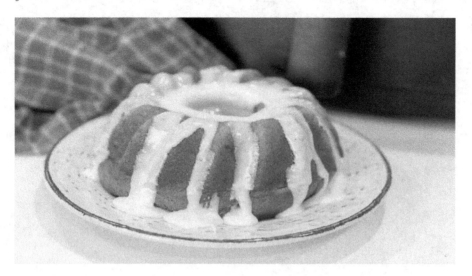

Cook time: 28 minutes

Serving: 8 people

Difficulty: Easy

Ingredients:

- 3/4 cup flour for all purposes

- 1/4 tbsp. salt

- 1 egg

- 2 mashed bananas overripe

- 1/4 cup sour cream

- 1/2 cup sugar

- 1/4 tbsp. baking soda

- 7-inch bundt pan

- 1/4 cup vegetable oil

- 1/2 tbsp. vanilla

Instructions:

1. In one tub, combine the dry ingredients and the wet ones in another. Mix the two slowly till flour is fully integrated, don't over mix.

2. With an anti-stick spray, spray and on a 7-inch bundt pan & then pour in the bowl.

3. Put it inside the air fryer basket & close. Placed it for 28 mins to 310 degrees

4. Remove when completed & permit to rest in the pan for about 5 mins.

5. When completed, detach and allow 5 minutes to sit in the pan. Then flip on a plate gently. Sprinkle melted icing on top, serve after slicing.

98. 3. Easy air fryer omelet

Cook time: 8 minutes

Serving: 2 people

Difficulty: Easy

Ingredients:

- 1/4 cup shredded cheese

- 2 eggs

- Pinch of salt

- 1 teaspoon of McCormick morning breakfast seasoning – garden herb

- Fresh meat & veggies, diced

- 1/4 cup milk

Instructions:

1. In a tiny tub, mix the milk and eggs till all of them are well mixed.

2. Add a little salt in the mixture of an egg.

3. Then, in the mixture of egg, add the veggies.

4. Pour the mixture of egg in a greased pan of 6 by 3 inches.

5. Place your pan inside the air fryer container.

6. Cook for about 8 to 10 mins and at 350 f.

7. While you are cooking, slather the breakfast seasoning over the eggs & slather the cheese on the top.

8. With a thin spoon, loose the omelet from the pan and pass it to a tray.

9. Loosen the omelet from the sides of the pan with a thin spatula and pass it to a tray.

10. Its options to garnish it with additional green onions.

99. 4. Air-fried breakfast bombs

Cook time: 20 mins

Serving: 2

Difficulty: easy

Ingredients:

• Cooking spray

• 1 tbsp. fresh chives chopped

• 3 lightly beaten, large eggs

• 4 ounces whole-wheat pizza dough freshly prepared

• 3 bacon slices center-cut

• 1 ounce 1/3-less-fat softened cream cheese

Instructions:

1. Cook the bacon in a standard size skillet for around 10 minutes, medium to very crisp. Take the bacon out of the pan; scatter. Add the eggs to the bacon drippings inside the pan; then cook, stirring constantly, around 1 minute, until almost firm and yet loose. Place the eggs in a bowl; add the cream cheese, the chives, and the crumbled bacon.

2. Divide the dough into four identical sections. Roll each bit into a five-inch circle on a thinly floured surface. Place a quarter of the egg mixture in the middle of each circle of dough. Clean the underside of the dough with the help of water; wrap the dough all around the mixture of an egg to form a purse and pinch the dough.

3. Put dough purses inside the air fryer basket in one layer; coat really well with the help of cooking spray. Cook for 5 to 6 minutes at 350 degrees f till it turns to a golden brown; check after 4 mins.

100.   5. Air fryer French toast

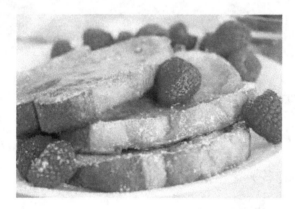

Cook time: 15 mins

Serving: 2 people

Difficulty: easy

Ingredients:

- 4 beaten eggs

- 4 slices of bread

- Cooking spray (non-stick)

Instructions:

1. Put the eggs inside a container or a bowl which is sufficient and big, so the pieces of bread will fit inside.

2. With a fork, mix the eggs and after that, place each bread slice over the mixture of an egg.

3. Turn the bread for one time so that every side is filled with a mixture of an egg.

4. After that, fold a big sheet of aluminum foil; this will keep the bread together. Switch the foil's side; this will ensure that the mixture of an egg may not get dry. Now put the foil basket in the air fryer basket. Make sure to allow space around the edges; this will let the circulation of hot air.

5. With the help of cooking spray, spray the surface of the foil basket and then put the bread over it. On top, you may add the excess mixture of an egg.

6. For 5 mins, place the time to 365 degrees f.

7. Turn the bread & cook it again for about 3 to 5 mins, until it's golden brown over the top of the French toast & the egg isn't runny.

8. Serve it hot, with toppings of your choice.

101.   6. Breakfast potatoes in the air fryer

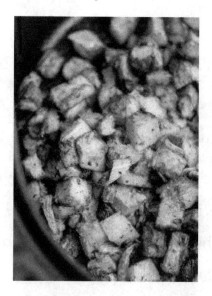

Cook time: 15 mins

Servings: 2

Difficulty: easy

Ingredients:

- 1/2 tbsp. kosher salt

- 1/2 tbsp. garlic powder

- Breakfast potato seasoning

- 1/2 tbsp. smoked paprika

- 1 tbsp. oil

- 5 potatoes medium-sized. Peeled & cut to one-inch cubes (Yukon gold works best)

- 1/4 tbsp. black ground pepper

Instructions:

1. At 400 degrees f, preheat the air fryer for around 2 to 3 minutes. Doing this will provide you the potatoes that are crispiest.

2. Besides that, brush your potatoes with oil and breakfast potato seasoning till it is fully coated.

3. Using a spray that's non-stick, spray on the air fryer. Add potatoes & cook for about 15 mins, shaking and stopping the basket for 2 to 3 times so that you can have better cooking.

4. Place it on a plate & serve it immediately.

102.   7. Air fryer breakfast pockets

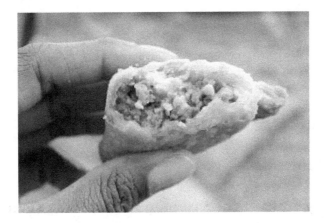

Cook time: 15 mins

Serving: 5 people

Difficulty: easy

Ingredients:

- 2-gallon zip lock bags

- Salt & pepper to taste

- 1/3 + 1/4 cup of whole milk

- 1 whole egg for egg wash

- Cooking spray

- 1-2 ounces of Velveeta cheese

- Parchment paper

- 1 lb. of ground pork

- 2 packages of Pillsbury pie crust

- 2 crusts to a package

- 4 whole eggs

Instructions:

1. Let the pie crusts out of the freezer.

2. Brown the pig and rinse it.

3. In a tiny pot, heat 1/4 cup of cheese and milk until it is melted.

4. Whisk four eggs, season with pepper and salt & add the rest of the milk.

5. Fumble the eggs in the pan until they are nearly fully cooked.

6. Mix the eggs, cheese and meat together.

7. Roll out the pie crust & cut it into a circle of about 3 to 4 inches (cereal bowl size).

8. Whisk 1 egg for making an egg wash.

9. Put around 2 tbsp. of the blend in the center of every circle.

10. Now, eggs wash the sides of the circle.

11. Create a moon shape by folding the circle.

12. With the help of a fork, folded edges must be crimped

13. Place the pockets inside parchment paper & put it inside a ziplock plastic bag overnight.

14. Preheat the air fryer for 360 degrees until it is ready to serve.

15. With a cooking spray, each pocket side must be sprayed.

16. Put pockets inside the preheated air fryer for around 15 mins or till they are golden brown.

17. Take it out from the air fryer & make sure it's cool before you serve it.

103.   8. Air fryer sausage breakfast casserole

Cook time: 20 mins

Serving: 6 people

Difficulty: easy

Ingredients:

- 1 diced red bell pepper

- 1 lb. ground breakfast sausage

- 4 eggs

- 1 diced green bell pepper

- 1/4 cup diced sweet onion

- 1 diced yellow bell pepper

- 1 lb. hash browns

Instructions:

1. Foil line your air fryer's basket.

2. At the bottom, put some hash browns.

3. Cover it with the raw sausage.

4. Place the onions & peppers uniformly on top.

5. Cook for 10 mins at 355 degrees.

6. Open your air fryer & blend the casserole a little if necessary.

7. Break every egg inside the bowl and spill it directly over the casserole.

8. Cook for the next 10 minutes for 355 degrees.

9. Serve with pepper and salt for taste.

104.   9. Breakfast egg rolls

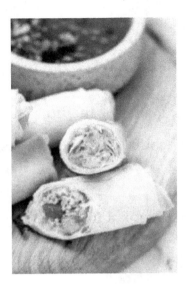

Cook time: 15 mins

Servings: 6 people

Difficulty: easy

Ingredients:

- Black pepper, to taste

- 6 large eggs

- Olive oil spray

- 2 tbsp. chopped green onions

- 1 tablespoon water

- 1/4 teaspoon kosher salt

- 2 tablespoons diced red bell pepper

- 1/2 pound turkey or chicken sausage

- 12 egg roll wrappers

- The salsa that is optional for dipping

Instructions:

1. Combine the water, salt and black pepper with the eggs.

2. Cook sausage in a non-stick skillet of medium size, make sure to let it cook in medium heat till there's no pink color left for 4 minutes, splitting into crumbles, then drain.

3. Stir in peppers and scallions & cook it for 2 minutes. Put it on a plate.

4. Over moderate flame, heat your skillet & spray it with oil.

5. Pour the egg mixture & cook stirring till the eggs are cooked and fluffy. Mix the sausage mixture.

6. Put one wrapped egg roll on a dry, clean work surface having corners aligned like it's a diamond.

7. Include an egg mixture of 1/4 cup on the lower third of your wrapper.

8. Gently raise the lower point closest to you & tie it around your filling.

9. Fold the right & left corners towards the middle & continue rolling into the compact cylinder.

10. Do this again with the leftover wrappers and fillings.

11. Spray oil on every side of your egg roll & rub it with hands to cover them evenly.

12. The air fryer must be preheated to 370 degrees f.

13. Cook the egg rolls for about 10 minutes in batches till it's crispy and golden brown.

14. Serve instantly with salsa, if required.

105.   10. Air fryer breakfast casserole

Cook time: 45 mins

Servings: 6 people

Difficulty: medium

Ingredients:

- 1 tbsp. extra virgin olive oil

- Salt and pepper

- 4 bacon rashers

- 1 tbsp. oregano

- 1 tbsp. garlic powder

- 2 bread rolls stale

- 1 tbsp. parsley

- 320 grams grated cheese

- 4 sweet potatoes of medium size

- 3 spring onions

- 8 pork sausages of medium size

- 11 large eggs

- 1 bell pepper

Instructions:

1. Dice and peel the sweet potato in cubes. Mix the garlic, salt, oregano and pepper in a bowl with olive oil of extra virgin.

2. In an air fryer, put your sweet potatoes. Dice the mixed peppers, cut the sausages in quarters & dice the bacon.

3. Add the peppers, bacon and sausages over the sweet potatoes. Air fry it at 160c or 320 f for 15 mins.

4. Cube and slice the bread when your air fryer is heating & pound your eggs in a blending jug with the eggs, including some extra parsley along with pepper and salt. Dice the spring onion.

5. Check the potatoes when you hear a beep from the air fryer. A fork is needed to check on the potatoes. If you are unable to, then cook for a further 2 to 3 minutes. Mix the basket of the air fryer, include the spring onions & then cook it for an additional five minutes with the same temperature and cooking time.

6. Using the projected baking pans, place the components of your air fryer on 2 of them. Mix it while adding bread and cheese. Add your mixture of egg on them & they are primed for the actual air fry.

7. Put the baking pan inside your air fryer & cook for 25 minutes for 160 c or 320 f. If you planned to cook 2, cook 1 first and then the other one. Place a cocktail stick into the middle & then it's done if it comes out clear and clean.

106.   11. Air fryer breakfast sausage ingredients

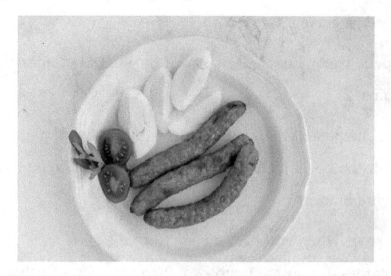

Cook time: 10 mins

Serving: 2 people

Difficulty: easy

Ingredients:

• 1 pound breakfast sausage

• Air fryer breakfast sausage ingredients

Instructions:

1. Insert your sausage links in the basket of an air fryer.

2. Cook your sausages or the sausage links for around 8 to 10 minutes at 360°.

107.   12. Wake up air fryer avocado boats

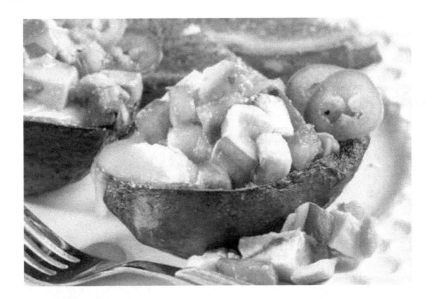

Cook time: 5 mins

Servings: 2

Difficulty: easy

Ingredients:

- 1/2 teaspoon salt

- 2 plum tomatoes, seeded & diced

- 1/4 teaspoon black pepper

- 1 tablespoon finely diced jalapeno (optional)

- 4 eggs (medium or large recommended)

- 1/4 cup diced red onion

- 2 avocados, halved & pitted

- 1 tablespoon lime juice

- 2 tablespoons chopped fresh cilantro

Instructions:

1. Squeeze the avocado fruit out from the skin with a spoon, leaving the shell preserved. Dice the avocado and put it in a bowl of medium-sized. Combine it with onion, jalapeno (if there is a need), tomato, pepper and cilantro. Refrigerate and cover the mixture of avocado until ready for usage.

2. Preheat the air-fryer for 350° f

3. Place the avocado shells on a ring made up of failing to make sure they don't rock when cooking. Just roll 2 three-inch-wide strips of aluminum foil into rope shapes to create them, and turn each one into a three-inch circle. In an air fryer basket, put every avocado shell over a foil frame. Break an egg in every avocado shell & air fry for 5 - 7 minutes or when needed.

4. Take it out from the basket; fill including avocado salsa & serve.

108.   12. Air fryer cinnamon rolls

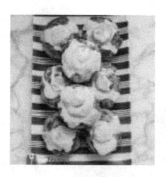

Cook time: 15 mins

Serving: 2 people

Difficulty: easy

Ingredients:

- 1 spray must non-stick cooking spray

- 1 can cinnamon rolls we used Pillsbury

Instructions:

1. put your cinnamon rolls inside your air fryer's basket, with the help of the rounds of 2. Parchment paper or by the cooking spray that is non-stick.

2. Cook at around 340 degrees f, 171 degrees for about 12 to 15 minutes, for one time.

3. Drizzle it with icing, place it on a plate and then serve.

109. 13. Air-fryer all-American breakfast dumplings

Cook: 10 minutes

Servings: 1 person

Difficulty: easy

Ingredients:

- Dash salt

- 1/2 cup (about four large) egg whites or liquid egg fat-free substitute

- 1 tbsp. Pre-cooked real crumbled bacon

- 1 wedge the laughing cow light creamy Swiss cheese (or 1 tbsp. reduced-fat cream cheese)

- 8 wonton wrappers or gyoza

Instructions:

1. By using a non-stick spray, spray your microwave-safe bowl or mug. Include egg whites or any substitute, salt and cheese wedge. Microwave it for around 1.5 minutes, mixing in between until cheese gets well mixed and melted and the egg is set.

2. Mix the bacon in. Let it cool completely for about 5 minutes.

3. Cover a wrapper of gyoza with the mixture of an egg (1 tablespoon). Moist the corners with water & fold it in half, having the filling. Tightly push the corners to seal. Repeat this step to make seven more dumplings. Make sure to use a non-stick spray for spraying.

4. Insert the dumplings inside your air fryer in one single layer. (Save the leftover for another round if they all can't fit). Adjust the temperature to 375 or the closest degree. Cook it for around 5 mins or till it's crispy and golden brown.

Chapter 2: Air fryer seafood recipe

110.   1. Air fryer 'shrimp boil'

Cook time: 15 mins

Servings: 2 people

Difficulty: easy

Ingredients:

- 2 tbsp. vegetable oil

- 1 lb. easy-peel defrosted shrimp

- 3 small red potatoes cut 1/2 inch rounds

- 1 tbsp. old bay seasoning

- 2 ears of corn cut into thirds

- 14 oz. smoked sausage, cut into three-inch pieces

Instructions:

1. Mix all the items altogether inside a huge tub & drizzle it with old bay seasoning, peppers, oil and salt. Switch to the air fryer basket attachment & place the basket over the pot.

2. Put inside your air fryer & adjust the setting of fish; make sure to flip after seven minutes.

3. Cautiously remove & then serve.

111.   2. Air fryer fish & chips

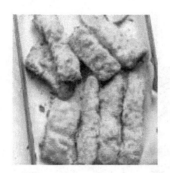

Cook time: 10 mins

Serving: 6 people

Difficulty: easy

Ingredients:

- Tartar sauce for serving

- ½ tbsp. garlic powder

- 1 pound cod fillet cut into strips

- Black pepper

- 2 cups panko breadcrumbs

- ½ cup all-purpose flour

- ¼ tbsp. salt

- Large egg beaten

- Lemon wedges for serving

- 2 teaspoons paprika

Instructions:

1. In a tiny tub, combine the flour, adding salt, paprika and garlic powder. Put your beaten egg in one bowl & your panko breadcrumbs in another bowl.

2. Wipe your fish dry with a towel. Dredge your fish with the mixture of flour, now the egg & gradually your panko breadcrumbs, pushing down gently till your crumbs stick. Spray both ends with oil.

3. Fry at 400 degrees f. Now turn halfway for around 10 to 12 mins until it's lightly brown and crispy.

4. Open your basket & search for preferred crispiness with the help of a fork to know if it easily flakes off. You may hold fish for an extra 1 to 2 mins as required.

5. Serve instantly with tartar sauce and fries, if required.

112.   3. Air-fryer scallops

Cook time: 20 mins

Servings: 2 people

Difficulty: easy

Ingredients:

- ¼ cup extra-virgin olive oil

- ½ tbsp. garlic finely chopped

- Cooking spray

- ½ teaspoons finely chopped garlic

- 8 large (1-oz.) Sea scallops, cleaned & patted very dry

- 1 tbsp. finely grated lemon zest

- ⅛ tbsp. salt

- 2 tbsps. Very finely chopped flat-leaf parsley

- 2 tbsp. capers, very finely chopped

- ¼ tbsp. ground pepper

Instructions:

1. Sprinkle the scallops with salt and pepper. Cover the air fryer basket by the cooking spray. Put your scallops inside the basket & cover them by the cooking spray. Put your basket inside the air fryer. Cook your scallops at a degree of 400 f till they attain the temperature of about 120 degrees f, which is an international temperature for 6 mins.

2. Mix capers, oil, garlic, lemon zest and parsley inside a tiny tub. Sprinkle over your scallops.

113.   4. Air fryer tilapia

Cook time: 6 mins

Servings: 4 people

Difficulty: easy

Ingredients:

- 1/2 tbsp. paprika

- 1 tbsp. salt

- 2 eggs

- 4 fillets of tilapia

- 1 tbsp. garlic powder

- 1/2 teaspoon black pepper

- 1/2 cup flour

- 2 tbsp. lemon zest

- 1 tbsp. garlic powder

- 4 ounces parmesan cheese, grated

Instructions:

1. Cover your tilapia fillets:

Arrange three deep dishes. Out of these, put flour in one. Blend egg in second and make sure that the eggs are whisked in the last dish mix lemon zest, cheese, pepper, paprika and salt. Ensure that the tilapia fillets are dry, and after that dip, every fillet inside the flour & covers every side. Dip into your egg wash & pass them for coating every side of the fillet to your cheese mixture.

2. Cook your tilapia:

Put a tiny sheet of parchment paper in your bask of air fryer and put 1 - 2 fillets inside the baskets. Cook at 400°f for around 4 - 5 minutes till the crust seems golden brown, and the cheese completely melts.

114. 5. Air fryer salmon

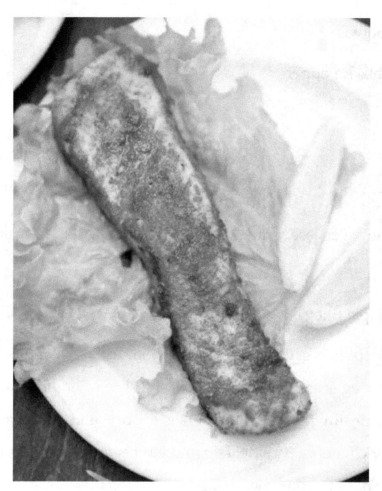

Cook time: 7 mins

Serving: 2 people

Difficulty: easy

Ingredients:

- 1/2 tbsp. salt

- 2 tbsp. olive oil

- 1/4 teaspoon ground black pepper

- 2 salmon fillets (about 1 1/2-inches thick)

- 1/2 teaspoon ginger powder

- 2 teaspoons smoked paprika

- 1 teaspoon onion powder

- 1/4 teaspoon red pepper flakes

- 1 tbsp. garlic powder

- 1 tablespoon brown sugar (optional)

Instructions:

1. Take the fish out of the refrigerator, check if there are any bones, & let it rest for 1 hour on the table.

2. Combine all the ingredients in a tub.

3. Apply olive oil in every fillet & then the dry rub solution.

4. Put the fillets in the Air Fryer basket.

5. set the air fryer for 7 minutes at the degree of 390 if your fillets have a thickness of 1-1/2-inches.

6. As soon as the timer stops, test fillets with a fork's help to ensure that they are ready to the perfect density. If you see that there is any need, then you cook it for a further few minutes. Your cooking time may vary with the temperature & size of the fish. It is best to set your air fryer for a minimum time, and then you may increase the time if there is a need. This will prevent the fish from being overcooked.

115.   6. Blackened fish tacos in the air fryer

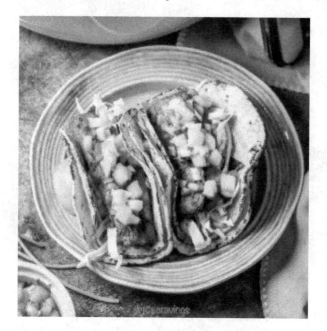

Cook time: 9 mins

Serving: 4 people

Difficulty: easy

Ingredients:

- 1 lb. Mahi mahi fillets (can use cod, catfish, tilapia or salmon)

- Cajun spices blend (or use 2-2.5 tbsp. store-bought Cajun spice blend)

- ¾ teaspoon salt

- 1 tbsp. paprika (regular, not smoked)

- 1 teaspoon oregano

- ½-¾ teaspoon cayenne (reduces or skips to preference)

- ½ teaspoon garlic powder

- ½ teaspoon onion powder

- ½ teaspoon black pepper

- 1 teaspoon brown sugar (skip for low-carb)

Additional ingredients for tacos:

- Mango salsa

- Shredded cabbage (optional)

- 8 corn tortillas

Instructions:

1. Get the fish ready

2. Mix cayenne, onion powder, brown sugar, salt, oregano, garlic powder, paprika and black pepper in a deep mixing tub.

3. Make sure to get the fish dry by using paper towels. Drizzle or brush the fish with a little amount of any cooking oil or olive oil. This allows the spices to stick to the fish.

4. Sprinkle your spice mix graciously on a single edge of your fish fillets. Rub the fish softly, so the ingredients stay on the fish.

5. Flip and brush the fish with oil on the other side & sprinkle with the leftover spices. Press the ingredients inside the fish softly.

6. Turn the air fryer on. Inside the basket put your fish fillets. Do not overlap the pan or overfill it. Close your basket.

7. Air fry the fish

8. Set your air fryer for 9 mins at 360°f. If you are using fillets which are thicker than an inch, then you must increase the cooking time to ten minutes. When the air fryer timer stops, with the help of a fish spatula or long tongs, remove your fish fillets.

9. Assembling the tacos

10. Heat the corn tortillas according to your preference. Conversely, roll them inside the towel made up of wet paper & heat them in the microwave for around 20 to 30 seconds.

11. Stack 2 small fillets or insert your fish fillet. Add a few tablespoons of your favorite mango salsa or condiment & cherish the scorched fish tacos.

12. Alternatively, one can include a few cabbages shredded inside the tacos & now add fish fillets on the top.

116.   7. Air fryer cod

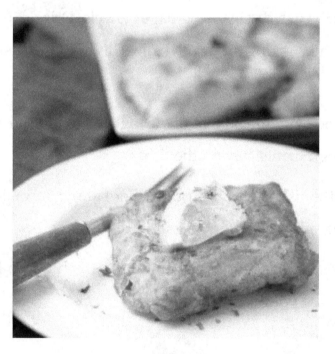

Cook time: 16 mins

Servings: 2 people

Difficulty: easy

Ingredients:

- 2 teaspoon of light oil for spraying

- 1 cup of plantain flour

- 0.25 teaspoon of salt

- 12 pieces of cod about 1 ½ pound

- 1 teaspoon of garlic powder

- 0.5 cup gluten-free flour blend

- 2 teaspoon of smoked paprika

- 4 teaspoons of Cajun seasoning or old bay

- Pepper to taste

Instructions:

1. Spray some oil on your air fryer basket & heat it up to 360° f.

2. Combine the ingredients in a tub & whisk them to blend. From your package, take the cod out and, with the help of a paper towel, pat dry.

3. Dunk every fish piece in the mixture of flour spice and flip it over & push down so that your fish can be coated.

4. Get the fish inside the basket of your air fryer. Ensure that there is room around every fish piece so that the air can flow round the fish.

5. Cook for around 8 minutes & open your air fryer so that you can flip your fish. Now cook another end for around 8 mins.

6. Now cherish the hot serving with lemon.

117.   8. Air fryer miso-glazed Chilean sea bass

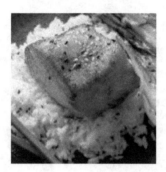

Cook time: 20 mins

Serving: 2 people

Difficulty: easy

Ingredients:

- 1/2 teaspoon ginger paste

- Fresh cracked pepper

- 1 tbsp. unsalted butter

- Olive oil for cooking

- 1 tbsp. rice wine vinegar

- 2 tbsp. miring

- 1/4 cup white miso paste

- 2 6 ounce Chilean sea bass fillets

- 4 tbsp. Maple syrup, honey works too.

Instructions:

1. Heat your air fryer to 375 degrees f. Apply olive oil onto every fish fillet and complete it with fresh pepper. Sprat olive oil on the pan of the air fryer and put the skin of the fish. Cook for about 12 to 15 minutes till you see the upper part change into golden brown color & the inner temperature now reached 135-degree f.

2. When the fish is getting cooked, you must have the butter melted inside a tiny saucepan in medium heat. When you notice that the butter melts, add maple syrup, ginger paste, miso paste, miring and rice wine vinegar, mix all of them till they are completely combined, boil them in a light flame and take the pan out instantly from the heat.

3. When your fish is completely done, brush the glaze and fish sides with the help of silicone pastry. Put it back inside your air fryer for around 1 to 2 extra minutes at 375 degrees f, till the glaze is caramelized. Complete it with green onion (sliced) & sesame seeds.

Instructions for oven

1. Heat the oven around 425 degrees f and put your baking sheet and foil sprayed with light olive oil. Bake it for about 20 to 25 minutes; this depends on how thick the fish is. The inner temperature must be around 130 degrees f when your fish is completely cooked.

2. Take out your fish, placed it in the oven & heat the broiler on a high flame. Now the fish must be brushed with miso glaze from the sides and the top & then put the fish inside the oven in the above rack. If the rack is very much near with your broiler, then place it a bit down, you might not want the fish to touch the broiler. Cook your fish for around 1 to 2 minutes above the broiler till you see it's getting caramelize. Make sure to keep a check on it as it happens very quickly. Complete it with the help of green onions (sliced) and sesame seeds.

118. 9. Air fryer fish tacos

Cook time: 35 mins

Serving: 6 people

Difficulty: Medium

Ingredients:

• ¼ teaspoon salt

• ¼ cup thinly sliced red onion

• 1 tbsp. water

• 2 tbsp. sour cream

• Sliced avocado, thinly sliced radishes, chopped fresh cilantro leaves and lime wedges

• 1 teaspoon lime juice

• ½ lb. skinless white fish fillets (such as halibut or mahi-mahi), cut into 1-inch strips

• 1 tbsp. mayonnaise

• 1 egg

• 1 package (12 bowls) old el Paso mini flour tortilla taco bowls, heated as directed on package

• 1 clove garlic, finely chopped

• ½ cup Progresso plain panko crispy bread crumbs

• 1 ½ cups shredded green cabbage

• 2 tbsp. old el Paso original taco seasoning mix (from 1-oz package)

Instructions:

1. Combine the sour cream, garlic, salt, mayonnaise and lime juice together in a medium pot. Add red onion and cabbage; flip to coat. Refrigerate and cover the mixture of cabbage until fit for serving.

2. Cut an 8-inch circle of parchment paper for frying. Place the basket at the bottom of the air fryer.

3. Place the taco-seasoning mix in a deep bowl. Beat the egg & water in another small bowl. Place the bread crumbs in another shallow dish. Coat the fish with your taco seasoning mix; dip inside the beaten egg, then cover with the mixture of bread crumbs, pressing to hold to it.

119. 10. Air fryer southern fried catfish

Cook time: 13 mins

Servings: 4 people

Difficulty: easy

Ingredients:

- 1 lemon

- 1/4 teaspoon cayenne pepper

- Cornmeal seasoning mix

- 1/4 teaspoon granulated onion powder

- 1/2 cup cornmeal

- 1/2 teaspoon kosher salt

- 1/4 teaspoon chili powder

- 2 pounds catfish fillets

- 1/4 teaspoon garlic powder

- 1 cup milk

- 1/4 cup all-purpose flour

- 1/4 teaspoon freshly ground black pepper

- 2 tbsp. dried parsley flakes

- 1/2 cup yellow mustard

Instructions:

1. Add milk and put the catfish in a flat dish.

2. Slice the lemon in two & squeeze around two tbsp. of juice added into milk so that the buttermilk can be made.

3. Place the dish in the refrigerator & leave it for 15 minutes to soak the fillets.

4. Combine the cornmeal-seasoning mixture in a small bowl.

5. Take the fillets out from the buttermilk & pat them dry with the help of paper towels.

6. Spread the mustard evenly on both sides of the fillets.

7. Dip every fillet into a mixture of cornmeal & coat well to create a dense coating.

8. Place the fillets in the greased basket of the air fryer. Spray gently with olive oil.

9. Cook for around 10 minutes at 390 to 400 degrees. Turn over the fillets & spray them with oil & cook for another 3 to 5 mins.

120.　11. Air fryer lobster tails with lemon butter

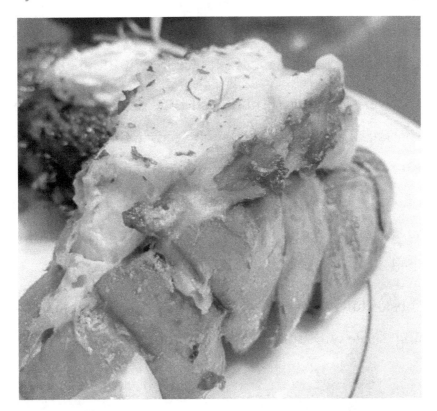

Cook time: 8 mins

Serving: 2 people

Difficulty: easy

Ingredients:

- 1 tbsp. fresh lemon juice

- 2 till 6 oz. Lobster tails, thawed

- Fresh chopped parsley for garnish (optional)

- 4 tbsp. melted salted butter

Instructions:

1. Make lemon butter combining lemon and melted butter. Mix properly & set aside.

2. Wash lobster tails & absorb the water with a paper towel. Butter your lobster tails by breaking the shell, take out the meat & place it over the shell.

3. Preheat the air fryer for around 5 minutes to 380 degrees. Place the ready lobster tails inside the basket of air fryer, drizzle with single tbsp. melted lemon butter on the meat of lobster. Cover the basket of the air fryer and cook for around 8 minutes at 380 degrees f, or when the lobster meat is not translucent. Open the air fryer halfway into the baking time, and then drizzle with extra lemon butter. Continue to bake until finished.

4. Remove the lobster tails carefully, garnish with crushed parsley if you want to, & plate. For dipping, serve with additional lemon butter.

121. 12. Air fryer crab cakes with spicy aioli + lemon vinaigrette

Cook time: 20 mins

Servings: 2 people

Difficulty: easy

Ingredients:

For the crab cakes:

- 1. Avocado oil spray

- 16-ounce lump crab meat

- 1 egg, lightly beaten

- 2 tbsp. finely chopped red or orange pepper

- 1 tbsp. Dijon mustard

- 2 tbsp. finely chopped green onion

- 1/4 teaspoon ground pepper

- 1/4 cup panko breadcrumbs

- 2 tbsp. olive oil mayonnaise

For the aioli:

- 1/4 teaspoon cayenne pepper

- 1/4 cup olive oil mayonnaise

- 1 teaspoon white wine vinegar

- 1 teaspoon minced shallots

- 1 teaspoon Dijon mustard

For the vinaigrette:

- 2 tbsp. extra virgin olive oil

- 1 tbsp. white wine vinegar

- 4 tbsp. fresh lemon juice, about 1 ½ lemon

- 1 teaspoon honey

- 1 teaspoon lemon zest

To serve:

- Balsamic glaze, to taste

- 2 cups of baby arugula

Instructions:

1. Make your crab cake. Mix red pepper, mayonnaise, ground pepper, crab meat, onion, panko and Dijon in a huge bowl. Make sure to mix the ingredients well. Then add eggs & mix the mixture again till it's mixed well. Take around 1/4 cup of the mixture of crab into cakes which are around 1 inch thick. Spray with avocado oil gently.

2. Cook your crab cakes. Organize crab cakes in one layer in the air fryer. It depends on the air fryer how many batches will be required to cook them. Cook for 10 minutes at 375 degrees f. Take it out from your air fryer & keep it warm. Do this again if required.

3. Make aioli. Combine shallots, Dijon, vinegar, cayenne pepper and mayo. Put aside for serving until ready.

4. Make the vinaigrette. Combine honey, white vinegar, and lemon zest and lemon juice in a ting jar. Include olive oil & mix it well until mixed together.

5. Now serve. Split your arugula into 2 plates. Garnish with crab cakes. Drizzle it with vinaigrette & aioli. Include few drizzles of balsamic glaze if desired.

Chapter 3: Air Fryer Meat and Beef recipe

122.   1. Air fryer steak

Cook time: 35 mins

Servings: 2

Difficulty: Medium

Ingredients:

- Freshly ground black pepper

- 1 tsp. freshly chopped chives

- 2 cloves garlic, minced

- 1(2 lb.) Bone-in rib eye

- 4 tbsp. Butter softened

- 1 tsp. Rosemary freshly chopped

- 2 tsp. Parsley freshly chopped

- 1 tsp. Thyme freshly chopped

- Kosher salt

Instructions:

1. In a tiny bowl, mix herbs and butter. Put a small layer of the wrap made up of plastic & roll in a log. Twist the ends altogether to make it refrigerate and tight till it gets hardened for around 20 minutes.

2. Season the steak with pepper and salt on every side.

3. Put the steak in the air-fryer basket & cook it around 400 degrees for 12 - 14 minutes, in medium temperature, depending on the thickness of the steak, tossing half-way through.

4. Cover your steak with the herb butter slice to serve.

123.   2. Air-fryer ground beef wellington

Cook time: 20 mins

Serving: 2 people

Difficulty: easy

Ingredients:

- 1 large egg yolk

- 1 tsp. dried parsley flakes

- 2 tsp. flour for all-purpose

- 1/2 cup fresh mushrooms chopped

- 1 tbsp. butter

- 1/2 pound of ground beef

- 1 lightly beaten, large egg, it's optional

- 1/4 tsp. of pepper, divided

- 1/4 tsp. of salt

- 1 tube (having 4 ounces) crescent rolls refrigerated

- 2 tbsp. onion finely chopped

- 1/2 cup of half & half cream

Instructions:

1. Preheat the fryer to 300 degrees. Heat the butter over a moderate flame in a saucepan. Include mushrooms; stir, and cook for 5-6 minutes, until tender. Add flour & 1/8 of a tsp. of pepper when mixed. Add cream steadily. Boil it; stir and cook until thickened, for about 2 minutes. Take it out from heat & make it aside.

2. Combine 2 tbsp. of mushroom sauce, 1/8 tsp. of the remaining pepper, onion and egg yolk in a tub. Crumble over the mixture of beef and blend properly. Shape it into two loaves. Unroll and divide the crescent dough into two rectangles; push the perforations to close. Put meatloaf over every rectangle. Bring together the sides and press to seal. Brush it with one beaten egg if necessary.

3. Place the wellingtons on the greased tray inside the basket of the air fryer in a single sheet. Cook till see the thermometer placed into the meatloaf measures 160 degrees, 18 to 22 minutes and until you see golden brown color.

Meanwhile, under low pressure, warm the leftover sauce; mix in the parsley. Serve your sauce, adding wellington.

124. 3. Air-fried burgers

Cook time: 10 mins

Serving: 4 people

Difficulty: easy

Ingredients:

- 500 g of raw ground beef (1 lb.)

- 1 tsp. of Maggi seasoning sauce

- 1/2 tsp. of ground black pepper

- 1 tsp. parsley (dried)

- Liquid smoke (some drops)

- 1/2 tsp. of salt (salt sub)

- 1 tbsp. of Worcestershire sauce

- 1/2 tsp. of onion powder

- 1/2 tsp. of garlic powder

Instructions:

1. Spray the above tray, and set it aside. You don't have to spray your basket if you are having an air fryer of basket-type. The cooking temperature for basket types will be around 180 c or 350 f.

2. Mix all the spice things together in a little tub, such as the sauce of Worcestershire and dried parsley.

2. In a huge bowl, add it inside the beef.

3. Mix properly, and make sure to overburden the meat as this contributes to hard burgers.

4. Divide the mixture of beef into four, & the patties are to be shape off. Place your indent in the middle with the thumb to keep the patties from scrunching up on the center.

5. Place tray in the air fry; gently spray the surfaces of patties.

6. Cook for around 10 minutes over medium heat (or more than that to see that your food is complete). You don't have to turn your patties.

7. Serve it hot on a pan with your array of side dishes.

125.   4. Air fryer meatloaf

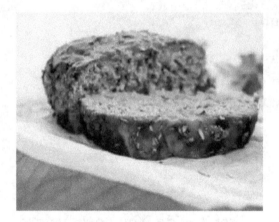

Cook time: 25 mins

Serving: 4 people

Difficulty: easy

Ingredients:

- 1/2 tsp. of Salt

- 1 tsp. of Worcestershire sauce

- 1/2 finely chopped, small onion

- 1 tbsp. of Yellow mustard

- 2 tbsp. of ketchup, divided

- 1 lb. Lean ground beef

- 1/2 tsp. Garlic powder

- 1/4 cup of dry breadcrumbs

- 1 egg, lightly beaten

- 1/4 tsp. Pepper

- 1 tsp. Italian seasoning

Instructions:

1. Put the onion, 1 tbsp. Ketchup, garlic powder, pepper, ground beef, egg, salt, breadcrumbs, Italian seasoning and Worcestershire sauce in a huge bowl.

2. Use hands to blend your spices with the meat equally, be careful you don't over-mix as it would make it difficult to over mix.

3. Shape meat having two inches height of 4 by 6, loaf. Switch your air fryer to a degree of 370 f & Put that loaf inside your air fryer.

4. Cook for fifteen min at a degree of 370 f.

5. In the meantime, mix the leftover 1 tbsp. of ketchup & the mustard in a tiny bowl.

6. Take the meatloaf out of the oven & spread the mixture of mustard over it.

7. Return the meatloaf to your air fryer & begin to bake at a degree of 370 degrees f till the thermometer placed inside the loaf measures 160 degrees f, around 8 to 10 further minutes.

8. Remove the basket from your air fryer when the meatloaf has touched 160 degrees f & then make the loaf stay inside the air fryer basket for around 5 to 10 minutes, after that slice your meatloaf.

126.   5. Air fryer hamburgers

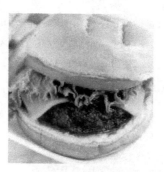

Cook time: 16 mins

Serving: 4 people

Difficulty: easy

Ingredients:

- 1 tsp. of onion powder

- 1 pound of ground beef (we are using 85/15)

- 4 pieces burger buns

- 1 tsp. salt

- 1/4 tsp. of black pepper

- 1 tsp. of garlic powder

- 1 tsp. of Worcestershire sauce

Instructions:

1. Method for standard ground beef:

2. Your air fryer must be preheated to 360 °.

3. In a bowl, put the unprocessed ground beef & add the seasonings.

4. To incorporate everything, make the of use your hands (or you can use a fork) & then shape the mixture in a ball shape (still inside the bowl).

5. Score the mixture of ground beef into 4 equal portions by having a + mark to split it.

Scoop out and turn each segment into a patty.

6. Place it in the air fryer, ensuring each patty has plenty of room to cook (make sure not to touch). If required, one can perform this in groups. We've got a bigger (5.8 quart) air fryer, and we did all of ours in a single batch.

7. Cook, turning half-way back, for 16 minutes. (Note: for bigger patties, you may have a need to cook longer.)

Process for Patties (pre-made):

1. In a tiny bowl, mix onion powder, pepper, garlic powder and salt, then stir till well mixed.

2. In a tiny bowl, pour in a few quantities of Worcestershire sauce. You may require A little more than one teaspoon (such as 1.5 tsp.), as some of it will adhere in your pastry brush.

3. Put patties on a tray & spoon or brush on a thin layer of your Worcestershire sauce.

4. Sprinkle with seasoning on every patty, saving 1/2 for another side.

5. With your hand, rub the seasoning to allow it to stick better.

6. Your air fryer should be preheated to 360 ° f.

7. Take out the basket when it's preheated & gently place your patties, seasoned one down, inside the basket.

8. Side 2 of the season, which is facing up the exact way as per above.

9. In an air fryer, put the basket back and cook for around 16 minutes, tossing midway through.

127.   6. Air Fryer Meatloaf

Cook time: 25 mins

Serving: 4 people

Difficulty: Easy

Ingredients:

• Ground black pepper for taste

• 1 tbsp. of olive oil, or as required

• 1 egg, lightly beaten

• 1 tsp. of salt

• 1 pound of lean ground beef

• 1 tbsp. fresh thyme chopped

• 3 tbsp. of dry bread crumbs

• 1 finely chopped, small onion

• 2 thickly sliced mushrooms

Instructions:

1. Preheat your air fryer to a degree of 392 f (200°C).

2. Mix together egg, onion, salt, ground beef, pepper, bread crumbs and thyme in a tub. 3. Thoroughly knead & mix.

4. Transfer the mixture of beef in your baking pan & smooth out the surface. The mushrooms are to be pressed from the top & coated with the olive oil. Put the pan inside the basket of the air fryer & slide it inside your air fryer.

5. Set the timer of the air fryer for around 25 minutes & roast the meatloaf till it is nicely browned.

6. Make sure that the meatloaf stays for a minimum of 10 minutes, and after that, you can slice and serve.

128.   7. Air Fryer Beef Kabobs

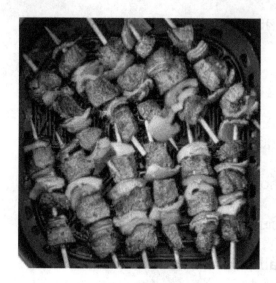

Cook time: 8 mins

Serving: 4 people

Difficulty: Easy

Ingredients:

- 1 big onion in red color or onion which you want

- 1.5 pounds of sirloin steak sliced into one-inch chunks

- 1 large bell pepper of your choice

For the marinade:

- 1 tbsp. of lemon juice

- Pinch of Salt & pepper

- 4 tbsp. of olive oil

- 1/2 tsp. of cumin

- 1/2 tsp. of chili powder

- 2 cloves garlic minced

Ingredients:

1. In a huge bowl, mix the beef & ingredients to marinade till fully mixed. Cover & marinate for around 30 minutes or up to 24 hours inside the fridge.

2. Preheat your air fryer to a degree of 400 f until prepared to cook. Thread the onion, pepper and beef onto skewers.

3. Put skewers inside the air fryer, which is already heated and the air fryer for about 8 to 10 minutes, rotating half-way until the outside is crispy and the inside is tender.

129.   8. Air-Fried Beef and Vegetable Skewers

Cook time: 8 mins

Serving: 2

Difficulty: easy

Ingredients:

- 2 tbs. of olive oil

- 2 tsp. of fresh cilantro chopped

- Kosher salt & freshly black pepper ground

- 1 tiny yellow summer squash, sliced into one inch (of 2.5-cm) pieces

- 1/4 tsp. of ground coriander

- Lemon wedges to serve (optional)

- 1/8 tsp. of red pepper flakes

- 1 garlic clove, minced

- 1/2 tsp. of ground cumin

- 1/2 yellow bell pepper, sliced into one inch (that's 2.5-cm) pieces

- 1/2 red bell pepper, sliced into one inch (that's 2.5-cm) pieces

- 1/2 lb. (that's 250 g) boneless sirloin, sliced into one inch (of 2.5-cm) cubes

- 1 tiny zucchini, sliced into one inch (that's 2.5-cm) pieces

- 1/2 red onion, sliced into one inch (that's 2.5-cm) pieces

Ingredients:

1. Preheat your air fryer at 390 degrees f (199-degree c).

2. In a tiny bowl, mix together one tablespoon of cumin, red pepper flakes and coriander. Sprinkle the mixture of spices generously over the meat.

3. In a tub, mix together zucchini, oil, cilantro, bell peppers, summer squash, cilantro, onion and garlic. Season with black pepper and salt to taste.

4. Tightly thread the vegetables and meat onto the four skewers adding two layers rack of air fryer, rotating the bits and equally splitting them. Put the skewers over the rack & carefully set your rack inside the cooking basket. Put the basket inside the air fryer. Cook, without covering it for around 7 - 8 minutes, till the vegetables are crispy and tender & your meat is having a medium-rare.

5. Move your skewers to a tray, and if you want, you can serve them with delicious lemon wedges.

130.   9. Air fryer taco calzones

Cook time: 10 mins

Serving: 2 people

Difficulty: easy

Ingredients:

• 1 cup of taco meat

• 1 tube of Pillsbury pizza dough thinly crust

• 1 cup of shredded cheddar

Instructions:

1. Spread out the layer of your pizza dough over a clean table. Slice the dough into four squares with the help of a pizza cutter.

2. By the use of a pizza cutter, cut every square into a big circle. Place the dough pieces aside to create chunks of sugary cinnamon.

3. Cover 1/2 of every dough circle with around 1/4 cup of taco meat & 1/4 cup of shredded cheese.

4. To seal it firmly, fold the remaining over the cheese and meat and push the sides of your dough along with the help of a fork so that it can be tightly sealed. Repeat for all 4 calzones.

5. Each calzone much is gently picked up & spray with olive oil or pan spray. Organize them inside the basket of Air Fryer.

Cook your calzones at a degree of 325 for almost 8 to 10 minutes. Monitor them carefully when it reaches to 8 min mark. This is done so that there is no chance of overcooking.

6. Using salsa & sour cream to serve.

7. For the making of cinnamon sugary chunks, split the dough pieces into pieces having equal sides of around 2 inches long. Put them inside the basket of the air fryer & cook it at a degree of 325 for around 5 minutes. Instantly mix with the one ratio four sugary cinnamon mixtures.

131. 10. Air Fryer Pot Roast

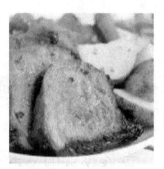

Cook time: 30 mins

Serving: 2 people

Difficulty: Medium

Ingredients:

- 1 tsp. of salt

- 3 tbsp. of brown sugar

- 1/2 cup of orange juice

- 1 tsp. of Worcestershire sauce

- 1/2 tsp. of pepper

- 3–4 pound thawed roast beef chuck roast

- 3 tbsp. of soy sauce

Instructions:

1. Combine brown sugar, Worcestershire sauce, soy sauce and orange juice.

2. Mix till the sugar is completely dissolved.

3. Spillover the roast & marinade for around 8 to 24 hours.

4. Put the roast in the basket of an air fryer.

5. Sprinkle the top with pepper and salt.

6. Air fry it at a degree of 400 f for around 30 minutes, turning it half-way through.

7. Allow it to pause for a period of 3 minutes.

8. Slice and serve into thick cuts.

Chapter 4: midnight snacks

132.   1. Air fryer onion rings

Cook time: 7 mins

Serving: 2 people

Difficulty: easy

Ingredients:

- 2 beaten, large eggs

- Marinara sauce for serving

- 1 ½ tsp. of kosher salt

- ½ tsp. of garlic powder

- 1 medium yellow onion, cut into half in about (1 1/4 cm)

- 1 cup of flour for all-purpose (125 g)

- 1 ½ cups of panko breadcrumbs (172 g)

- 1 tsp. of paprika

- ⅛ tsp. of cayenne

- ½ tsp. of onion powder

- ½ tsp. black pepper freshly ground

Instructions:

1. Preheat your air fryer to 190°c (375°f).

2. Use a medium-size bowl to mix together onion powder, salt, paprika, cayenne, pepper, flour and garlic powder.

3. In 2 separate small cups, add your panko & eggs.

4. Cover onion rings with flour, then with the eggs, and afterward with the panko.

Working in lots, put your onion rings in one layer inside your air fryer & "fry" for 5 to 7 minutes or till you see golden brown color.

5. Using warm marinara sauce to serve.

133.   2. Air fryer sweet potato chips

Cook time: 15 mins

Serving: 2

Difficulty: easy

Ingredients:

- 1 ½ tsp. of kosher salt

- 1 tsp. of dried thyme

- 1 large yam or sweet potato

- ½ tsp. of pepper

- 1 tbsp. of olive oil

Instructions:

1. Preheat your air fryer to a degree of 350 f (180 c).

2. Slice your sweet potato have a length of 3- to 6-mm (1/8-1/4-inch). In a medium tub, mix your olive oil with slices of sweet potato until well-seasoned. Add some pepper, thyme and salt to cover.

3. Working in groups, add your chips in one sheet & fry for around 14 minutes till you see a golden brown color and slightly crisp.

Fun.

134.   3. Air fryer tortilla chips

Cook time: 5 mins

Serving: 2 people

Difficulty: easy

Ingredients:

- 1 tbsp. of olive oil

- Guacamole for serving

- 2 tsp. of kosher salt

- 12 corn of tortillas

- 1 tbsp. of McCormick delicious jazzy spice blend

Instructions:

1. Preheat your air fryer at a degree of 350 f (180 c).

2. Gently rub your tortillas with olive oil on every side.

3. Sprinkle your tortillas with delicious jazzy spice and salt mix on every side.

Slice every tortilla into six wedges.

4. Functioning in groups, add your tortilla wedges inside your air fryer in one layer & fry it for around 5 minutes or until you see golden brown color and crispy texture.

Serve adding guacamole

135. 4. Air fryer zesty chicken wings

Cook time: 20 mins

Serving: 2 people

Difficulty: easy

Ingredients:

- 1 ½ tsp. of kosher salt

- 1 ½ lb. of patted dry chicken wings (of 680 g)

- 1 tbsp. of the delicious, zesty spice blend

Instructions:

1. Preheat your air fryer at 190°c (375°f).

2. In a tub, get your chicken wings mixed in salt & delicious zesty spice, which must be blend till well-seasoned.

3. Working in lots, add your chicken wings inside the air fryer in one layer & fry it for almost 20 minutes, turning it halfway through.

4. Serve it warm

136. 5. Air fryer sweet potato fries

Cook time: 15 mins

Serving: 2 people

Difficulty: easy

Ingredients:

- 1/4 tsp. of sea salt

- 1 tbsp. of olive oil

- 2 (having 6-oz.) sweet potatoes, cut & peeled into sticks of 1/4-inch

- Cooking spray

- 1/4 tsp. of garlic powder

- 1 tsp. fresh thyme chopped

Instructions:

1. Mix together thyme, garlic powder, olive oil and salt in a bowl. Put sweet potato inside the mixture and mix well to cover.

2. Coat the basket of the air fryer gently with the help of cooking spray. Place your sweet potatoes in one layer inside the basket & cook in groups at a degree of 400 f until soft inside & finely browned from outside for around 14 minutes, rotating the fries halfway through the cooking process.

137. 6. Air fryer churros with chocolate sauce

Cook time: 30 mins

Serving: 12

Difficulty: easy

Ingredients:

• 1/4 cup, adding 2 tbsp. Unsalted butter that's divided into half-cup (around 2 1/8 oz.)

• 3 tbsp. of heavy cream

• Half cup water

• 4 ounces of bitter and sweet finely chopped baking chocolate

• Flour for All-purpose

• 2 tsp. of ground cinnamon

• 2 large eggs

• 1/4 tsp. of kosher salt

• 2 tbsp. of vanilla kefir

• 1/3 cup of granulated sugar

Instruction:

1. Bring salt, water & 1/4 cup butter and boil it in a tiny saucepan with a medium-high flame. Decrease the heat to around medium-low flame; add flour & mix actively with a spoon made up of wood for around 30 seconds.

2. Stir and cook continuously till the dough is smooth. Do this till you see your dough continues to fall away from the sides of the pan & a film appears on the bottom of the pan after 2 to 3 minutes. Move the dough in a medium-sized bowl. Stir continuously for around 1 minute until slightly cooled. Add one egg from time to time while stirring continuously till you see it gets smoother after every addition. Move the mixture in the piping bag, which is fitted with having star tip of medium size. Chill it for around 30 minutes.

3. Pipe 6 (3" long) bits in one-layer inside a basket of the air fryer. Cook at a degree of 380 f for around 10 minutes. Repeat this step for the leftover dough.

4. Stir the sugar & cinnamon together inside a medium-size bowl. Use 2 tablespoons of melted butter to brush the cooked churros. Cover them with the sugar mixture.

5. Put the cream and chocolate in a tiny, microwaveable tub. Microwave with a high temperature for roughly 30 seconds until molten and flat, stirring every 15 seconds. Mix in kefir.

6. Serve the churros, including chocolate sauce.

138.   7. Whole-wheat pizzas in an air fryer

Cook time: 10 mins

Serving: 2 people

Difficulty: easy

Ingredients:

• 1 small thinly sliced garlic clove

• 1/4 ounce of Parmigiano-Reggiano shaved cheese (1 tbsp.)

- 1 cup of small spinach leaves (around 1 oz.)

- 1/4 cup marinara sauce (lower-sodium)

- 1-ounce part-skim pre-shredded mozzarella cheese (1/4 cup)

- 1 tiny plum tomato, sliced into 8 pieces

- 2 pita rounds of whole-wheat

Instructions:

1. Disperse marinara sauce equally on one side of every pita bread. Cover it each with half of the tomato slices, cheese, spinach leaves and garlic.

2. Put 1 pita in the basket of air-fryer & cook it at a degree of 350 f until the cheese is melted and the pita is crispy. Repeat with the leftover pita.

139.   8. Air-fried corn dog bites

Cook time: 15 mins

Serving: 4 people

Difficulty: easy

Ingredients:

- 2 lightly beaten large eggs

- 2 uncured hot dogs of all-beef

- Cooking spray

- 12 bamboo skewers or craft sticks

- 8 tsp. of yellow mustard

- 1 1/2 cups cornflakes cereal finely crushed

- 1/2 cup (2 1/8 oz.) Flour for All-purpose

Instructions:

1. Split lengthwise every hot dog. Cut every half in three same pieces. Add a bamboo skewer or the craft stick inside the end of every hot dog piece.

2. Put flour in a bowl. Put slightly beaten eggs in another shallow bowl. Put crushed cornflakes inside another shallow bowl. Mix the hot dogs with flour; make sure to shake the surplus. Soak in the egg, helping you in dripping off every excess. Dredge inside the cornflakes crumbs, pushing to stick.

3. Gently coat the basket of the air fryer with your cooking spray. Put around six bites of corn dog inside the basket; spray the surface lightly with the help of cooking spray. Now cook at a degree of 375 f till the coating shows a golden brown color and is crunchy for about 10 minutes, flipping the bites of corn dog halfway in cooking. Do this step with other bites of the corn dog.

4. Put three bites of corn dog with 2 tsp. of mustard on each plate to, and then serve immediately.

140. 9. Crispy veggie quesadillas in an air fryer

Cook time: 20 mins

Serving: 4 people

Difficulty: easy

Instructions:

- Cooking spray

- 1/2 cup refrigerated and drained pico de gallo

- 4 ounces far educing cheddar sharp cheese, shredded (1 cup)

- 1 tbsp. of fresh juice (with 1 lime)

- 4(6-in.) whole-grain Sprouted flour tortillas

- 1/4 tsp. ground cumin

- 2 tbsp. fresh cilantro chopped

- 1 cup red bell pepper sliced

- 1 cup of drained & rinsed black beans canned, no-salt-added

- 1 tsp. of lime zest plus

- 1 cup of sliced zucchini

- 2 ounces of plain 2 percent fat reduced Greek yogurt

Instructions:

1. Put tortillas on the surface of your work. Sprinkle two tbsp. Shredded cheese on the half of every tortilla. Each tortilla must be top with cheese, having a cup of 1/4 each black beans, slices of red pepper equally and zucchini slices. Sprinkle equally with the leftover 1/2 cup of cheese. Fold the tortillas making a shape of a half-moon. Coat quesadillas lightly with the help of cooking spray & protect them with toothpicks.

2. Gently spray the cooking spray on the basket of the air fryer. Cautiously put two quesadillas inside the basket & cook it at a degree of 400 f till the tortillas are of golden brown color & slightly crispy, vegetables get softened, and the cheese if finally melted for around 10 minutes, rotating the quesadillas halfway while cooking. Do this step again with the leftover quesadillas.

3. As the quesadillas are cooking, mix lime zest, cumin, yogurt and lime juice altogether in a small tub. For serving, cut the quesadilla in slices & sprinkle it with cilantro. Serve it with a tablespoon of cumin cream and around 2 tablespoons of pico de gallo.

141.   10. Air-fried curry chickpeas

Cook time: 10 mins

Serving: 4 people

Difficulty: easy

Ingredients:

- 2 tbsp. of curry powder

- Fresh cilantro thinly sliced

- 1(15-oz.) Can chickpeas (like garbanzo beans), rinsed & drained (1 1/2 cups)

- 1/4 tsp. of kosher salt

- 1/2 tbsp. of ground turmeric

- 1/2 tsp. of Aleppo pepper

- 1/4 tsp. of ground coriander

- 2 tbsp. of olive oil

- 1/4 tsp. and 1/8 tsp. of Ground cinnamon

- 2 tbsp. of vinegar (red wine)

- 1/4 tsp. of ground cumin

Instructions:

1. Smash chickpeas softly inside a tub with your hands (don't crush); remove chickpea skins.

2. Apply oil and vinegar to chickpeas, & toss for coating. Add turmeric, cinnamon, cumin, curry powder and coriander; whisk gently so that they can be mixed together.

3. Put chickpeas in one layer inside the bask of air fryer & cook at a degree of 400 f till it's crispy for around 15 mins; shake the chickpeas timely while cooking.

4. Place the chickpeas in a tub. Sprinkle it with cilantro, Aleppo pepper and salt; blend to coat.

142.   11. Air fry shrimp spring rolls with sweet chili sauce.

Cook time: 20 mins

Serving: 4

Difficulty: easy

Ingredients:

• 1 cup of matchstick carrots

• 8 (8" square) wrappers of spring roll

• 2 1/2 tbsp. of divided sesame oil

• 4 ounces of peeled, deveined and chopped raw shrimp

• 1/2 cup of chili sauce (sweet)

• 1 cup of (red) bell pepper julienne-cut

- 2 tsp. of fish sauce

- 3/4 cup snow peas julienne-cut

- 2 cups of cabbage, pre-shredded

- 1/4 tsp. of red pepper, crushed

- 1 tbsp. of lime juice (fresh)

- 1/4 cup of fresh cilantro (chopped)

Instructions:

1. In a large pan, heat around 1 1/2 tsp. of oil until softly smoked. Add carrots, bell pepper and cabbage; Cook, stirring constantly, for 1 to 1 1/2 minutes, until finely wilted. Place it on a baking tray; cool for 5 minutes.

2. In a wide tub, place the mixture of cabbage, snow peas, cilantro, fish sauce, red pepper, shrimp and lime juice; toss to blend.

3. Put the wrappers of spring roll on the surface with a corner that is facing you. Add a filling of 1/4 cup in the middle of every wrapper of spring roll, extending from left-hand side to right in a three-inch wide strip.

4. Fold each wrapper's bottom corner over the filling, stuffing the corner tip under the filling. Fold the corners left & right over the filling. Brush the remaining corner softly with water; roll closely against the remaining corner; press gently to cover. Use 2 teaspoons of the remaining oil to rub the spring rolls.

5. Inside the basket of air fryer, put four spring rolls & cook at a degree of 390 f till it's golden, for 6 - 7 minutes, rotating the spring rolls every 5 minutes. Repeat with the leftover spring rolls. Use chili sauce to serve.

Chapter 5: Dessert recipes

143. 1. Air fryer mores

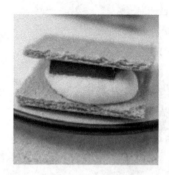

Cook time: 2 mins

Serving: 2 people

Difficulty: easy

Ingredients:

- 1 big marshmallow

- 2 graham crackers split in half

- 2 square, fine quality chocolate

Instructions:

1. Preheat the air fryer at a degree of 330 f.

2. When preheating, break 2 graham crackers into two to form four squares. Cut 1 big marshmallow into half evenly so that one side can be sticky.

3. Add every half of your marshmallow in a square of one graham cracker & push downwards to stick the marshmallow with graham cracker. You must now have two marshmallows coated with graham crackers & two regular graham crackers.

4. In one layer, put two graham crackers and marshmallows inside your air fryer & cook for about 2 minutes till you can see the marshmallow becoming toasted slightly.

5. Remove immediately and completely and add 1 chocolate square to the toasted marshmallow. Add the rest of the squares of the graham cracker and press down. Enjoy instantly.

144.   2. Easy air fryer brownies

Cook time: 15 mins

Serving: 4 people

Difficulty: easy

Ingredients:

- 2 large eggs

- ½ cup flour for all-purpose

- ¼ cup melted unsalted butter

- 6 tbsp. of cocoa powder, unsweetened

- ¼ tsp. of baking powder

- ¾ cup of sugar

- ½ tsp. of vanilla extract

- 1 tbsp. of vegetable oil

- ¼ tsp. of salt

Instructions:

1. Get the 7-inch baking tray ready by gently greasing it with butter on all the sides and even the bottom. Put it aside

2. Preheat the air fryer by adjusting its temperature to a degree of 330 f & leaving it for around 5 minutes as you cook the brownie batter.

3. Add baking powder, cocoa powder, vanilla extract, flour for all-purpose, butter, vegetable oil, salt, eggs and sugar in a big tub & mix it unless well combined.

4. Add up all these for the preparation of the baking pan & clean the top.

5. Put it inside the air fryer & bake it for about 15 minutes or as long as a toothpick can be entered and comes out easily from the center.

6. Take it out and make it cool in the tray until you remove and cut.

145.   3. Easy air fryer churros

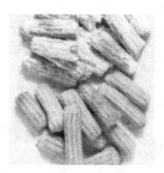

Cook time: 5 mins

Serving: 4 people

Difficulty: easy

Ingredients:

- 1 tbsp. of sugar

- Sifted powdered sugar & cinnamon or cinnamon sugar

- 1 cup (about 250ml) water

- 4 eggs

- ½ cup (113g) butter

- ¼ tsp. salt

- 1 cup (120g) all-purpose flour

Instructions:

1. Mix the ingredients bringing them to boil while stirring continuously.

2. Add flour & start mixing properly. Take it out from the heat & mix it till it gets smooth & the dough can be taken out from the pan easily.

3. Add one egg at one time and stir it until it gets smooth. Set it to cool.

4. Preheat your air fryer degree of 400 for 200 c.

5. Cover your bag of cake decorations with dough & add a star tip of 1/2 inch.

6. Make sticks which are having a length of 3 to 4 inches by moving your dough out from the bag in paper (parchment). You can now switch it inside your air fryer if you are ready to do so. If it is hard to handle the dough, put it inside the refrigerator for around 30 minutes.

7. Use cooking spray or coconut oil to spray the tray or the basket of your air fryer.

8. Add around 8 to 10 churros in a tray or inside the basket of the air fryer. Spray with oil.

9. Cook for 5 minutes at a degree of 400 for 200 c.

10. Until finished and when still hot, rill in regular sugar, cinnamon or sugar mixture.

11. Roll in the cinnamon-sugar blend, cinnamon or normal sugar until finished and when still high.

146.   4. Air fryer sweet apples

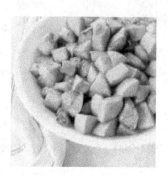

Cook time: 8 mins

Serving: 4 people

Difficulty: easy

Ingredients:

- ¼ cup of white sugar

- ⅓ Cup of water

- ¼ cup of brown sugar

- ½ tsp. of ground cinnamon

- 6 apples diced and cored

- ¼ tsp. of pumpkin pie spice

- ¼ tsp. of ground cloves

Instructions:

1. Put all the ingredients in a bowl that is oven safe & combine it with water and seasonings. Put the bowl inside the basket, oven tray or even in the toaster of an air fryer.

2. Air fry the mixture of apples at a degree of 350 f for around 6 minutes. Mix the apples & cook them for an extra 2 minutes. Serve it hot and enjoy.

147.   5. Air fryer pear crisp for two

Cook time: 20 mins

Serving: 2

Difficulty: easy

Ingredients:

- ¾ tsp. of divided ground cinnamon

- 1 tbsp. of softened salted butter

- 1 tsp. of lemon juice

- 2 pears. Peeled, diced and cored

- 1 tbsp. of flour for all-purpose

- 2 tbsp. of quick-cooking oats

- 1 tbsp. of brown sugar

Instructions:

1. Your air fryer should be preheated at a degree of 360 f (180 c).

2. Mix lemon juice, 1/4 tsp. Cinnamon and pears in a bowl. Turn for coating and then split the mixture into 2 ramekins.

3. Combine brown sugar, oats, leftover cinnamon and flour in the tub. Using your fork to blend in the melted butter until the mixture is mushy. Sprinkle the pears.

4. Put your ramekins inside the basket of an air fryer & cook till the pears become bubbling and soft for around 18 - 20 minutes.

148.   6. Keto chocolate cake – air fryer recipe

Cook time: 10 mins

Serving: 6 people

Difficulty: easy

Ingredients:

- 1 tsp. of vanilla extract

- 1/2 cup of powdered Swerve

- 1/3 cup of cocoa powder unsweetened

- 1/4 tsp. of salt

- 1 & 1/2 cups of almond flour

- 2 large eggs

- 1/3 cups of almond milk, unsweetened

- 1 tsp. of baking powder

Instructions:

1. In a big mixing tub, mix every ingredient until they all are well mixed.

2. Butter or spray your desired baking dish. We used bunt tins in mini size, but you can even get a 6-inch cake pan in the baskets of the air fryer.

3. Scoop batter equally inside your baking dish or dishes.

4. Set the temperature of the air fryer to a degree of 350 f & set a 10-minute timer. Your cake will be ready when the toothpick you entered comes out clear and clean.

Conclusion:

The air fryer seems to be a wonderful appliance that will assist you with maintaining your diet. You will also enjoy the flavor despite eating high amounts of oil if you prefer deep-fried food.

Using a limited quantity of oil, you will enjoy crunchy & crispy food without the additional adverse risk, which tastes exactly like fried food. Besides, the system is safe & easy to use. All you must do is choose the ingredients needed, and there will be nutritious food available for your family.

An air fryer could be something which must be considered if a person is attempting to eat a diet having a lower-fat diet, access to using the system to prepare a range of foods, & want trouble cooking experience.